ADAPTIVE DISCLOSURE

Also Available

Early Intervention for Trauma and Traumatic Loss
Edited by Brett T. Litz

ADAPTIVE DISCLOSURE

A New Treatment for Military Trauma, Loss, and Moral Injury

Brett T. Litz,
Leslie Lebowitz, Matt J. Gray,
and William P. Nash

THE GUILFORD PRESS
New York   London

The authors have checked with sources believed to be reliable in their efforts to provide
information that is complete and generally in accord with the standards of practice that are
accepted at the time of publication. However, in view of the possibility of human error or
changes in behavioral, mental health, or medical sciences, neither the authors, nor the editors
and publisher, nor any other party who has been involved in the preparation or publication
of this work warrants that the information contained herein is in every respect accurate or
complete, and they are not responsible for any errors or omissions or the results obtained from
the use of such information. Readers are encouraged to confirm the information contained in
this book with other sources.

The views and opinions expressed in this volume are those of the authors, alone,
and do not necessarily reflect the official policies of the Departments of Defense
or Veterans Affairs or the United States Marine Corps.

Library of Congress Cataloging-in-Publication Data

Names: Litz, Brett T.
Title: Adaptive disclosure : a new treatment for military trauma, loss, and moral injury / by Brett
  T. Litz [and four others].
Description: New York : The Guilford Press, 2016. | Includes bibliographical references and index.
Identifiers: LCCN 2015037307 | ISBN 9781462523290 (hardback) | ISBN 9781462533831 (paperback)
Subjects: LCSH: Post-traumatic stress disorder—Treatment. | Veterans—Mental health. | Psychic
  trauma—Treatment. | War—Psychological aspects.
  BISAC: PSYCHOLOGY / Psychopathology / Post-Traumatic Stress Disorder
  (PTSD). | MEDICAL / Psychiatry / General. | SOCIAL SCIENCE / Social Work.
  | PSYCHOLOGY / Psychotherapy / Counseling. | MEDICAL / Nursing / Psychiatric.
Classification: LCC RC552.P67 L58 2015 | DDC 616.85/21—dc23
LC record available at http://lccn.loc.gov/2015037307

About the Authors

Brett T. Litz, PhD, is Professor in the Departments of Psychiatry and Psychology at Boston University and Director of the Mental Health Core of the Massachusetts Veterans Epidemiological Research and Information Center at the VA Boston Healthcare System. He is also Assessment Core Director of the STRONG STAR Consortium and the Consortium to Alleviate PTSD. Dr. Litz focuses on evaluating the mental health outcomes associated with military deployments across the lifespan, with an emphasis on early intervention and treatments for combat and operational trauma, loss, and moral injury.

Leslie Lebowitz, PhD, is a clinical psychologist in private practice in Newton Center, Massachusetts. She consults extensively in forensic contexts and provides training in the area of trauma in both community and military settings. Dr. Lebowitz developed the psychological portion of the curriculum for training Air Force Sexual Assault Response Coordinators and continues to do biannual training for the Air Force. Her research focuses on the psychological meaning of trauma and the implications for treatment. Previous research examined the aftermath of sexual violence, and more recent work addresses traumatic loss and moral injury.

Matt J. Gray, PhD, is Professor of Psychology at the University of Wyoming. His research and publications focus on treatment development for broad emotional and psychological impacts of combat, as well as prevention and treatment of sexual violence and intimate partner violence. Dr. Gray has received the Extraordinary Merit in Research Award and the Outstanding Psychology Faculty Member Award on multiple occasions from the University of Wyoming.

William P. Nash, MD, is Director of Psychological Health for the U.S. Marine Corps. While on active duty in the Navy, Dr. Nash was deployed to Iraq with Marines of the 1st Marine Division during the Second Battle of Fallujah. His current interests focus on the prevention, recognition, and treatment of combat and operational stress injuries, including moral injury. He is coeditor of *Combat Stress Injuries: Theory, Research, and Management* and founding chair of the Military Committee of the Group for the Advancement of Psychiatry.

Preface

This book offers a new psychotherapy framework to help service members and veterans heal from war-related psychological, spiritual, biological, and social injuries. We call this new approach "adaptive disclosure." Adaptive disclosure originated from a call from the Department of Defense in 2007 for each military branch to generate novel stress-reduction and resilience-promoting intervention strategies for active duty service members. Accordingly, Bill Nash, then a Navy Captain heading Combat and Operational Stress Control (COSC) for the Navy and Marine Corps, asked Brett Litz to generate an innovative approach that fit deployed service members' lived experience, was consistent with the Navy and Marine Corps model of COSC (a doctrine authored by Nash in collaboration with Marine Corps leaders), and took into account the three principal harms of war specified in the COSC doctrine: traumatic loss, life-threat trauma, and serious ethical and moral transgressions ("moral injury").

Thus, the original adaptive disclosure project was a program evaluation funded by the Navy. The funding allowed us time to develop the approach, write a treatment manual, and conduct an open trial at Marine Corps Base Camp Pendleton. Brett Litz assembled a team to generate the treatment manual and to train and supervise the therapists for the pilot project. Two expert trauma therapists and scholars, Leslie Lebowitz and Matt Gray, helped write the original manual. Bill, Leslie, and Matt helped to concretize, synthesize, and systematize the nascent therapy model. They also helped to provide rich, poignant, and clinically lively procedural heuristics and guides to helping service members and veterans using adaptive disclosure strategies.

We leveraged the positive initial results from the open trial (Gray et al., 2012; Steenkamp et al., 2011) to obtain funding from the Congressionally Directed Medical Research Program in the Department of Defense (award number W81XWH-10-1-0810) to conduct a randomized controlled trial of adaptive disclosure, again in the Marine Corps at Camp Pendleton, comparing adaptive disclosure with cognitive processing therapy. This trial is ongoing as of the writing of this book, inviting a legitimate question: why not wait until the efficacy trial is finished to share adaptive disclosure? Our reasoning is the following: First, we receive many requests for the manual and invitations to consult about adaptive disclosure. The impression we all have is that clinicians in the military and the U.S. Department of Veterans Affairs (VA) are hungry for an approach that formally targets loss and, especially, moral injury. Second, although we think adaptive disclosure should be applied as we describe it in the book, namely as a planned series of sessions with specific foci, we also designed the book to help clinicians conceptualize war trauma cases idiographically and dimensionally, to equip them to fully appreciate the military ethos and use that understanding clinically, and to allow clinicians who use other approaches to extract practical procedural strategies to help service members and veterans with prolonged grief from loss and moral injury.

This therapy guide is intended for clinicians of any discipline tasked with helping service members and veterans heal and recover from various war wounds. We trust it will be useful for civilian and uniformed mental health professionals within and outside the military (and VA), as well as chaplains and medical providers. We also hope researchers may glimpse frontiers for research for the promotion of mental health in individuals and groups affected by war. Care providers trained or certified to conduct evidence-based cognitive-behavioral therapies, such as prolonged exposure and cognitive processing therapy, will be well prepared to apply adaptive disclosure (or specific strategies in the model) to augment their work with service members or veterans.

ACKNOWLEDGMENTS

Brett T. Litz: Adaptive disclosure stems from the intellectual collaboration, friendship, and reciprocal mentoring of Bill Nash, an active duty psychiatrist who had deployed to war to care for Marines, and myself that started around 2005. For me, this meeting of the minds could not have been more fortunate or well timed. Because I had been collaborating with military partners in various research endeavors in the military context, I had a vantage point that few trauma professionals in the VA and civilian settings have. I was learning to be more circumspect, curious, and humble about the extent to which the current thinking about trauma and evidence-based treatment models, chiefly derived from civilian trauma or work in the VA far removed from the military context, fit the early needs of service members in situ. Bill helped me to recognize and embrace what I did not know, which, although disquieting, allowed me to be open and curious about what needed to be done to best help our service members and veterans. Bill also helped mentor me to become more personal and emotionally engaged with service members and their experiences. He helped me bond with military caregivers and he helped provide opportunities to listen to service members. These experiences created a sense of purpose and commitment to helping service members, families, and, consequently, veterans suffering from the various mental wounds of war.

Both Bill and I were also especially keen on countering the zeitgeist in the posttraumatic stress disorder (PTSD) field, which emphasizes danger and threat experiences as necessary and sufficient to explain the etiology and maintenance of PTSD, as well as the treatment needs of war veterans. We wanted not only to generate a model of psychotherapy that was consistent with our emerging understanding of war trauma but also to build an approach that fostered, as a necessity, a respect for and understanding of the military culture and ethos. We knew the field needed an approach that could be disseminated among care providers who are unfamiliar with the military, one that required compassion and understanding. The chapter on the military culture, written solely by Bill, offers readers a perspective that is fundamental to adaptive disclosure.

Adaptive disclosure therapy and this book would not be possible without the collaboration and friendship of Ariel Lang, who was a principal investigator in our open trial of adaptive disclosure. Ariel helped train and supervise the therapists at Camp Pendleton, and she helped conduct the program evaluation. Amy Amidon, Amy Lansing, and Alex Laifer were extraordinary psychotherapists who learned and applied the model and helped us learn as we fielded the therapy. Adaptive disclosure would not exist were it not for the Navy and Marine Corps, which supported our work, and the patient and loyal Marines with PTSD who allowed us to try to help them. Finally, a thank you to Jennifer Wortmann, who provided excellent feedback and helped edit several chapters.

Leslie Lebowitz: I have spent my professional life studying and treating traumatized people. When people are traumatized, they are driven to understand and create meaning out of their experience, and the conclusions they draw have the power to reconstruct their perceptions of themselves, other people, and the rules of life. My interests have centered on these meanings, how they can either injure or heal, and how they can be changed. The study of psychological trauma has also compelled me, allowing me to touch on broad social concerns through the intimate process of psychotherapy. The experience of being a part of a society in near continual warfare without in any way addressing this ongoing tragedy has left me feeling uncomfortably and unconscionably disconnected. I was therefore enormously grateful and honored to join this team and have the opportunity to contribute, in some way, to ameliorating the ongoing anguish emanating from these wars.

Many writers have defined trauma as too much of an unbearable reality (Jonathan Shay calls it the too much "muchness" of trauma), and this is certainly true of war. There is no way to minimize, sanitize, or not be changed by what one learns in the context of combat, and there is no way to heal without engaging with the thoughts and feelings one desperately and understandably wants to avoid. Grappling with these thoughts and feelings in a manner that is respectful, collaborative, and active defines adaptive disclosure.

Our intention has been to create an intervention that uses the heat of traumatic emotion to engender new learning, potent enough to alter traumatic meanings. We started from a humble and respectful posture of genuine curiosity—asking what meaning this event has for this person and where he or she is caught within that understanding. The imperative to meet people where they were most injured led us to create multiple therapeutic options so that we could address the divergent ways individuals construct their experiences. We pulled freely from techniques and perspectives that are derived from different traditions, including dynamic, cognitive, behavioral, mindfulness, and Gestalt therapies. Grounding and shaping all of this work was the necessity to respect and incorporate the military context: its challenges, structures, culture, strengths, and vulnerabilities.

A trauma perspective locates reality in the center of the therapeutic and theoretical discourse. While inter- and intrapersonal dynamics, the ever-present and active unconscious, and the inexorable need to have and create meaning all press on the task of understanding an individual in pain, in adaptive disclosure, the work returns, again and again, to the problem of learning to accept and tolerate a complex and difficult reality. For example, when considering moral injury and its related guilt and sense of responsibility, rather than a blanket assumption that self-blame is always defensive or neurotic, we ask the question: Where does responsibility reasonably lie and what can and should be done about it? Similarly, in discussions of grief, we ask: What has really been lost, in the other person, in one's life-sustaining ideals and values, in one's notions about oneself? Throughout, we engage the task of repair as needing to occur within the individual, within the therapy hour and therapeutic relationship, and through actions taken in the world.

It was an amazing team. Brett Litz created and managed a collaboration that kept us anchored to the task of creating a systematic, emotionally intense, safe, respectful therapeutic process capable of modifying the original traumatic experience. The veterans' unique needs always came first, even within the demands of a protocol-based model. Brett engendered a sense of wide-open creative inquiry that capitalized on the team members' strengths and wove together our disparate perspectives with great skill. Bill Nash brought a profound and essential understanding of military culture and the experience of combat, as well as a lifetime of work, engaging deeply, soulfully, and unflinchingly with people who have endured almost unbearable horror. Matt Gray brought a calm clarity to the writing and to the difficult process of structuring and systematizing the therapeutic work. The clinicians (Amy Lansing, Amy Amidon, and Alex Laifer) were intrepid. They marched into heartbreakingly painful and complex material with warmth, commitment, creativity, and compassion. Their insights and suggestions consistently enhanced the work.

The treatment had startling effects for such a short-term intervention given that it was up against what was often catastrophic, complex trauma. Adaptive disclosure underscores that direct engagement with traumatic injury, in conjunction with an understanding of the social context, facilitates trust (as compared to needing trust to develop relationally in order to engage traumatic pain). It not only led clients to a new understanding of what had happened, but also introduced them to a process that may well provide some inoculation against future isolation and despair. In this sense, it is as much a seed-planting technique as a reparative one, which is valuable given that complex trauma and its harms tend to unfold over the course of development.

The technique cuts to the chase while incorporating the varied ways in which individuals interpret their experiences, and it offers a therapeutic process to address these critical idiosyncratic meanings systematically. To my mind, it incorporates the best of cognitive-behavioral therapy (evidence based, direct, active, targeted) and the best of exposure (approaching and working with painful, threatening emotions directly), weaving these together with disparate therapeutic approaches designed to facilitate change within this population.

It is our hope that the techniques described in this book will inform the work of clinicians seeking to help veterans and ease some of the pain caused by these wars.

Matt J. Gray: I have long been interested in cognitive appraisals of traumatic event exposure and the consequences that they have for posttraumatic adjustment. Much of my clinical and research work to date has centered on meanings that survivors extract from their experiences and the profound implications that disparate interpretations of an event can have for recovery. Though I was trained in conventional, best-practice therapies for trauma treatment and have used these interventions extensively, I began to appreciate that particular types of clinical presentations were less responsive to these treatments. Specifically, individuals experiencing sudden and profound loss, those whose appraisals—though intensely distressing—were not altogether irrational or errant, and those who had fundamentally altered perceptions of self (i.e., moral injury) as a result of their experiences tended not to improve to the same degree as those trauma survivors presenting with more conventional fear- and anxiety-based symptoms, or whose cognitions were in fact misplaced (e.g., self-blame following sexual assault). These observations can easily be dismissed as yet another instance of erroneous clinical intuition, but not as easily swept aside is the empirical literature demonstrating nontrivial attrition, substantive residual distress, and recidivism associated with even our best treatments (for a review, see Steenkamp & Litz, 2013).

These observations and the search for—and subsequent development of—an alternative approach to treating varied combat stress injuries need not be taken as an indictment of established trauma treatment approaches. It is not necessary to be an exclusive adherent of either prolonged exposure (PE) or cognitive processing therapy (CPT) on the one hand, or adaptive disclosure or other emergent treatments on the other. As with most disorders and variants of distress, even our best treatments leave considerable room for improvement. We certainly can and should use those interventions where appropriate, and in my own clinical work, I continue to use PE and CPT extensively for individuals presenting primarily with fear- and anxiety-based responding, and for those likely to benefit from conventional cognitive restructuring to target erroneous beliefs. It is not necessary or productive to "choose sides," and this certainly was not our intent when embarking on the adaptive disclosure project. Rather than trying to supplant established treatments, we attempted to consider and to develop promising techniques to address common consequences of combat that do not lend themselves as readily to standard frameworks.

Scientifically minded and research-informed clinicians have an ethical mandate to continue to develop novel treatments and enhance existing ones in an effort to improve on current clinical outcomes. Some efforts will "move the ball forward" and others will fail. But it would be most unfortunate and unwise to assume that we are at an endpoint where treatment development is concerned—and this is true of every domain of psychopathology. All too often, a "best-practice" moniker is inappropriately used to justify a moratorium on treatment development efforts or the consideration of alternative approaches. If we are to meet the clinical needs of our patients and clients, continuing to develop and rigorously evaluate new approaches is essential. It would be difficult indeed to make a cogent case that we are anywhere near an endpoint in treatment development based on the proportion of patients who do not respond to current best-practice treatments, as well as those exhibiting considerable residual distress following treatment.

Clinicians working with veteran and military populations have long appreciated that some patients are haunted by regret for their actions or inactions in combat. Quite often, these appraisals are indeed inaccurate and overgeneralized. Rather than being truly culpable for unfortunate outcomes, the patients in question are afflicted by hindsight bias (mistaking what they now know to be true for what they possibly could have known at the time) or counterfactual thinking (retrospectively thinking about all of the decisions and actions that could have altered the outcome—but, here again, based on present knowledge, not what was known at the time). Conventional cognitive restructuring and reappraisal techniques work quite well in these instances. Yet there are others who volitionally and knowingly engaged in questionable acts that violated their moral codes. Attempting to challenge the veracity of their appraisals or to dismiss them as owing to the fog of war is likely to be unproductive. Similarly, it is our opinion that helping military personnel move forward when suffering the loss of a fallen comrade requires an approach other than that used to address fear- and anxiety-based PTSD presentations.

I am especially grateful to Brett Litz for inviting me to join him in this endeavor. His clinical insights and wisdom, coupled with my intrinsic interests in narrative and meaning-making approaches to address diverse emotional sequelae of trauma, made this an especially attractive project for me. I have benefited tremendously from the collective wisdom and clinical skill of the entire adaptive disclosure team, including (but not limited to) Bill Nash, Leslie Lebowitz, Ariel Lang, and Amy Amidon. Much empirical work remains to be done, but we hope this approach will be useful to therapists who struggle, as we did, with treatment considerations for moral injury and traumatic loss. Much more importantly, we hope the approach described here proves to be beneficial for veterans and military personnel who are struggling with these problems. These issues are complex and can be overwhelming, but it is our firm belief that they are not insurmountable, and we hope that adaptive disclosure provides a promising path forward.

William P. Nash: I don't know whether the whole world changed on September 11, 2001, as some claim, but I know for sure my world was forever changed by the events of that day, only not all at once. At the time, I was practicing psychiatry as an active duty naval officer at the hospital on Camp Pendleton in southern California, the home of roughly one-third of the Marine Corps' total fighting forces. Prior to September 11, 2001, my practice included a broad spectrum of mental disorders and life problem challenges in Marines, sailors, service members, veterans, and their family members, ranging from schizophrenia in the young to dementia in the old, including many problems arising from acute or chronic stress. After that day, I spent my days increasingly listening to the heart-wrenching stories of service members who had survived the attacks on the Pentagon and the World Trade Center, or who had participated in subsequent search and recovery operations. Once the wars in Afghanistan and Iraq got rolling, my clinical practice became exclusively involved in the treatment of combat-related PTSD in otherwise healthy and successful young service members.

I was stunned. As a military psychiatrist who had cut his teeth on Vietnam veterans in the 1980s, many of them still serving on active duty, I thought I knew something about combat-related PTSD. I didn't. Acute trauma, I learned, was as different from chronic trauma as day from night. And everything I thought I knew about risk factors was proven incomplete, if not downright wrong, by the healthy and heroic, highly trained, and expertly led young men and women who repeatedly proved to me that everyone has a breaking point.

In January 2004, I left clinical practice to train with the 1st Marine Division as it prepared to relieve the Army's hard-hit 82nd Airborne Division in the Al Anbar Province of Iraq. My uncertainties about the treatment of combat-related PTSD paled in comparison to my feelings of utter inadequacy in trying to prevent psychological wounds in a war zone. What a tremendous gift the Marines and leaders of the 1st Marine Division gave me as they invited me to join their world, to see the mind-boggling challenges of urban, counterinsurgency warfare through their eyes, and to feel the relief of success and the pain of failure and loss through their hearts. I will be forever grateful to two of the best (and most patient) teachers I may ever have: Colonel Willy Buhl and Colonel Pat Malay, commanding officers of 3rd Battalion, 1st Marines, and 3rd Battalion, 5th Marines, during the Battle of Fallujah in November 2004.

After I returned from Iraq, I was invited by Lieutenant General Pete Osman, deputy commandant responsible for all Marine manpower and wellness efforts, to transfer to Headquarters, Marine Corps, to help develop their combat and operational stress control programs. His sponsorship and trust made everything that followed possible. Knowing I had little chance to succeed in my new job without a lot of help from someone smarter than I in the academic world, one of my first acts after arriving in Quantico, Virginia, in late 2005, was to introduce myself on the phone to Brett Litz. What a blessing Brett has been to me personally and professionally ever since. In our partnership, we have found growing common ground for diverse aspects of our professional identities: psychiatrist and psychologist, service member and VA professional, researcher and boots-on-the-ground clinician. In our efforts to invite reconsideration in both our cultures of time-honored but questionable assumptions, Brett Litz and I have truly been brothers in arms.

I recall the phone call in 2007, in which Brett told me about his idea for adaptive disclosure. It was immediately clear to me that what he proposed would fill a need to combine evidence-based and culturally sensitive aspects of care into one treatment for combat-related PTSD. I soon met and began collaboration with Leslie Lebowitz and Matt Gray, who have contributed loving hearts and clear intellect to this important project. The therapists we found for our pilot project and randomized controlled trial—Amy Amidon, Amy Lansing, and Alex Laifer—are all gifted clinicians. Anyone reading this book should consider tracking them down to learn more about how to actually do adaptive disclosure. Ariel Lang, at VA San Diego, has led our Department of Defense–funded randomized clinical trial masterfully and, for all of us working on it, painlessly.

As I write this, the Institute of Medicine's Committee on the Assessment of Ongoing Efforts in the Treatment of PTSD is completing its final report on the prevention, screening, and treatment of PTSD across the Department of Defense and the VA. As a member of this committee, I have been fortunate to participate in vigorous discussions cutting to the heart of the challenge of reducing the psychological burdens of war on service members, veterans, and our communities. I now take the liberty of anticipating a few of the Committee's findings. First, after reviewing reams of literature and visiting dozens of military bases and VA health care centers, it has become crystal clear that no one has yet found the "magic bullet" for combat-related PTSD. It simply does not yet exist. Given the great heterogeneity of PTSD, and its chronicity beyond a certain point, as well as the many ways in which the lives of those with persistent symptoms are bent by their ongoing distress and limitations in functioning, it seems unlikely that a singular, broadly effective treatment will ever be found. Second, although fear-conditioning conceptions of PTSD will always enjoy relevance and validity, PTSD is not always and only about fear. The gauntlet has been thrown for basic science researchers to develop animal models for the higher cortical components of PTSD, such as complicated loss and moral injury. Finally, what has helped members of various military and civilian populations recover from posttraumatic stress has always been some combination of the same core elements, the same ones clearly identified by systematic reviews and clinical practice guidelines: retelling and reprocessing, making meaning, and relearning the world. Adaptive disclosure aims to deliver these elements in the language and culture of the warfighter, for whom we have the greatest respect and gratitude.

Contents

Purchasers of this book can download and
print enlarged versions of Appendices 2 and 3
at *www.guilford.com/litz2-forms* for personal use
or use with individual clients.

CHAPTER 1

Introduction

In this book, we describe the background, rationale, and procedures for "adaptive disclosure," a novel treatment approach for war trauma developed specifically for active duty service members and veterans (Gray et al., 2012; Steenkamp et al., 2011). The aim of adaptive disclosure is to help service members and veterans recover and heal from combat stress injuries and posttraumatic stress disorder (PTSD). It promotes coming to terms with the meaning and implication of the three core types of traumatic war experiences (life threat, loss, moral injury) and reduction of damaging ways of construing their long-term impact.

A key assumption of adaptive disclosure is that dangerous combat and operational experiences such as life threats that elicit fear are not the only source of psychic injury during warfare. This supposition runs counter to the central and often exclusive role that life-threatening trauma and the fear-conditioning model play in extant conceptualizations of the mental and behavioral health consequences of war trauma, chiefly PTSD and the treatment needs of service members and war veterans. Indeed, this state of affairs has been codified in the newest iteration of the PTSD construct (American Psychiatric Association, 2013). In the *Diagnostic and Statistical Manual of Mental Disorders*, Fifth Edition (DSM-5), the only stressor necessary for PTSD entails experiences with death, life-threat, and actual or threatened serious injury (including sexual violence). Although in DSM-5, PTSD is technically no longer classified as an anxiety disorder, it remains a condition that is danger- and threat-based.

1

Conceptually, adaptive disclosure stems from our belief that family members, service members, clinicians, and communities need to appreciate that dangerous life-threatening experiences in war are not the only potential source of mental, physical, and spiritual injury for combatants. Because of training, professionalism, leadership, support, and the military culture and ethos, dangerous combat experiences may actually not be traumatizing for many service members and may be the least impactful for many veterans over the lifespan. Unlike civilian traumatic event contexts, there is good reason to assume that most threat-based stress reactions are mitigated by military preselection and tough and realistic training and preparation, and, when present, are healed by indigenous military rituals and assets. For example, peer and social supports, subsequent training and preparation, and effective leadership are arguably sufficient to recover from high-danger experiences. There are systematic opportunities for service members exposed to war zone dangers to get respite, unburden, and vent their thoughts and feelings about the experience, and strengthen bonds and derive meaning from the experience by sharing narratives about danger—all of which are resonant with the warrior culture and ideal. In learning theory terms, leaders in the theater of operations typically ensure sufficient exposure to high-fear contexts to provide natural extinction of conditioned fear and exposure to corrective mastery experiences that thwart the development of problematic schemas (beliefs) about safety and control. Even when service members develop a life-threat-based stress injury in theater, arguably the most pressing problem is not high states of fear and arousal, but rather the self-condemnation and guilt that may arise from letting peers and leaders down because of a perceived or real temporary incapacitation in the field. If indigenous mechanisms of recovery are inadequate to resolve danger-based sequelae, conventional exposure-based therapies are likely to be highly effective (Foa, Keane, Friedman, & Cohen, 2008). In contrast to danger-based experiences, there are arguably fewer indigenous military resources to prepare for traumatic loss and to promote resilience and recovery in the face of loss of life (especially the survivor guilt that can ensue; see Pivar & Field, 2004). There are even fewer resources to mitigate and heal the lasting impact of perpetrating, failing to prevent, or bearing witness to war zone acts that produce inner conflict because of moral compromise, that is, "moral injury."

Adaptive disclosure is unique because it employs cognitive-behavioral therapy (CBT) and other therapeutic strategies to target not only life-threatening trauma, but also traumatic loss (and attendant guilt), and inner conflict produced by moral injury associated with shame and self-handicapping behaviors (Litz et al., 2009; Stein et al., 2012). Adaptive disclosure is designed to help service members and veterans experientially and emotionally process these divergent types of war zone harms, traumas, and losses. The goal is to help service members and veterans gain exposure to corrective and more productive ways of construing the implications of diverse war experiences in terms of their military (or newly found civilian) identity, how they feel about themselves, how they relate to other people, and how they construct a narrative about their future. The assumption is that each of the three war-related principal harms depicted in Table 1.1 entails distinct peri-event reactions, phenomenologies, and unfolding need states and motivations, as shown in this table, and downstream behavioral, psychological, biological, and spiritual impacts (Litz, Steenkamp, & Nash, 2014).

In adaptive disclosure, we ask the question "What do service members and veterans need to heal and recover from the three different harms?" The answer to this question guides the choice of change agents in the therapy.

At the start of the therapy, service members or veterans identify a military experience that is currently haunting and consuming them. This experience is categorized as a *life-threatening event*, a *traumatic loss*, or a *moral injury*. At its core, adaptive disclosure entails exposure-based, experiential and emotion-focused processing of this principal combat or operational experience and a real-time rendering of constructions

TABLE 1.1. Distinguishing Elements of the Three Principal Harms

| | Event type | | |
	Life threat	Loss	Moral injury
Peri-event reactions	Fear, horror, helplessness, panic, dissociation	Sadness (or numbness), rage, shock, anguish	Guilt, shame, rage
Phenomenology	Anxiety, stress, conditioned emotional response	Withdrawal, guilt, haunted	Unforgiven, self-handicapping, anomie
Unfolding need and corrective elements	Safety, mastery, confidence	Reconnection, reengagement	Forgiveness, compassion

about the implications of the event in terms of self-view, professional role (especially if on active duty), expectations about others, and the future. For all trauma types, as with other CBT-based approaches, adaptive disclosure provides a sober but hopeful, evocative, and emotion-focused opportunity for service members and veterans to realize how they have changed as a result of combat and operational experiences, to think about who they want to be, and to get a sense of how to get there experientially. Unlike other CBT for PTSD, adaptive disclosure individualizes treatment for service members with PTSD by employing different strategies to target danger-, loss-, and moral injury-based principal war zone harms.

Life-threatening or danger-focused harms lead to generalized expectancies of future harms and dangers. The needs that arise from intensely horrifying experiences are validation and understanding from others about the legitimacy and universality of vulnerability; comfort; and the expectation of safety, self-control, mastery, and competence. For life-threatening harms, exposure therapies, principally prolonged exposure (PE), are the treatments of choice on conceptual and empirical grounds (Foa et al., 2008). Consequently, the approach to life-threatening harm in adaptive disclosure is similar to that in PE. For events that are loss-related or morally injurious, separate breakout strategies are used to foster exposure to corrective experience and new learning specific to these dynamics.

The unique needs that arise from attachment loss vary with the quality and dependency of the relationship and whether the loss is unexpected, and especially, whether it is due to violence. If a service member or veteran is haunted by a war-related loss, it is safe to assume that the relationship was powerful, that it was due to violence or a tragic circumstance of some kind, and that the person may feel responsible in some way or feel guilty about surviving. The needs that are acquired over time are successful connection and reconnection with healthy and positive attachments, reengagement in pleasurable activities and wellness behaviors, self-forgiveness, and finding ways of paying respect and honoring the lost person. For loss, after an exposure component, which entails raw emotional processing of the loss and a disclosure of unfiltered thoughts about the meaning and implication of the loss (usually self-blame and guilt), adaptive disclosure entails a dialogue in imagination with the lost friend. The aim is for the patient to acknowledge the loss's impact and meaning in real time to the lost friend, then also to voice what the friend says about this in real time. The goal is to promote an emotionally charged accommodation of the corrective "messages" voiced by the friend who would only want the patient to live well.

If a service member or veteran seeking treatment for putative PTSD endorses a moral and ethical transgression, especially an act of perpetration, he or she is likely to be consumed by shame and guilt, struggle with feelings of unworthiness and anomie, and may be self-handicapping and potentially self-harming (Litz et al., 2009). Needless to say, these experiences are uniquely tarnishing and toxic. The needs that are accessible and at the forefront for patients are antithetical to, and perhaps negate, healing—namely, to suffer, to be punished, and to be unforgiven. What we should infer is that there are deeper needs to be forgiven in order to have self-compassion, and to correct, to make amends. Ideally, service members and veterans recommit to prior values and belief systems and can identify a path forward—a path based on the knowledge that a regrettable action need not be destiny. In adaptive disclosure, we attempt to expose patients to *corrective* learning experiences that counter harm-specific self- and other-expectations. Rather than focusing on (exclusively) reliving a morally injurious event or helping the patient dispute the accuracy of beliefs implicated by the event (as is done in other CBT), one of the main change agents in adaptive disclosure to redress moral injury is an evocative imaginal "confession" and dialogue with a compassionate and forgiving moral authority in order to begin to challenge and address the shame and self-handicapping that accompany such experiences. There are also homework assignments to begin the process of being exposed to goodness, repairing by giving back, and so forth. The assumption of adaptive disclosure is that the treatment starts, but cannot finish, the moral repair process. The goal is not to attempt to eradicate or fully replace self-constructions of moral compromise; this would be impossible. The goal is to foster balance. Adaptive disclosure attempts to help patients accept the part of themselves that did or was subjected to bad acts, without attempting to modify constructions about culpability and the moral implications of the events. At the same time, the therapy is designed to help patients reclaim goodness and humanity, and to have those parts manifested in their lives, we hope, as prominently as possible. Ultimately, the expectation is that self-forgiveness and accommodating the possibility of also living a moral and virtuous life requires life course changes for most veterans of war.

Implementing adaptive disclosure requires clinicians to have a firm grasp and understanding of the military ethos and culture. In addition to providing a background and rationale for the treatment approach, it is our hope that this book will educate care providers about military values and identity as a platform from which to understand the presentation of a patient and the goals of treatment. The book is designed to help care providers across disciplines (social workers, counselors, psychologists, psychiatrists) in any context (in and outside the Departments of Veterans Affairs and Defense facilities) learn and apply the therapy to service members and veterans who need help recovering and healing from various combat and operational experiences. The book is also designed to educate care providers about the military culture and ethos, military trauma, loss, and moral injury, and to be prepared to help service members who report having problems that stem from loss and moral injury in whatever model of care they use.

BACKGROUND

Approximately 10–20% of the 2 million U.S. troops who have served in the wars in Afghanistan and Iraq experience significant mental health difficulties including PTSD, depression, and anxiety (e.g., Hoge et al., 2004; see Litz & Schlenger, 2009). Because PTSD and other mental and behavioral health problems among veterans of war are pernicious and disabling (e.g., Dohrenwend et al., 2006; Kulka et al., 1990; Prigerson, Maciejewski, & Rosenheck, 2001), a major public health challenge is to redress military trauma-related problems as early as possible and to prevent spiraling dysfunction, suffering, premature discharge, and chronic problems over the life course (see Litz & Bryant, 2009).

While limited, evidence-based mental health treatment such as CBT may be available to some service members in theater (see Cigrang, Peterson, & Schobitz, 2005). For most service members, the most viable and prudent time to provide early treatment is postdeployment, while they are in garrison (at their home base). However, during this time, service members are busy with demanding training regimens and preparations for subsequent deployments that absorb a good deal of attention and mental effort. Consequently, service members' needs and availability for care differ from those of patients receiving trauma-focused CBT in civilian and veteran outpatient settings. Not only is service members' time limited but also their inclination to focus on emotional and psychological matters is constrained by the understandable need (and social and occupational pressures) to "carry on."

Although there is ample evidence that CBT strategies such as PE and *cognitive processing therapy* (CPT) are effective PTSD treatments among civilian motor vehicle accident and sexual assault survivors (see Foa et al., 2008), these approaches have been shown to be *substantially less efficacious* with complex military trauma (e.g., Rauch et al., 2009; Ready et al., 2008; Schnurr et al., 2007; see Steenkamp & Litz, 2013). We argue that this is the case for at least two reasons, each of which we have tried to redress in the adaptive disclosure approach.

Many care providers in the military and the U.S. Department of Veterans Affairs (VA) have not adequately considered the unique cultural and contextual elements of military trauma, the phenomenology of service members' lived experience, or the clinical issues that arise from combat and operational stressors, such as traumatic loss and experiences that are morally compromising. Too often clinicians assume that life-threatening war zone experiences are necessary and sufficient to explain their patients' experiences and what requires redressing in therapy. They are at risk for failing to realize the contribution of military features, such as leader actions or the quality of connections to unit members. Furthermore, in our opinion, there are significant missing elements in the current CBT care models with respect to treating war trauma.

When considering possible limitations in the application of current CBT treatment models, several factors become apparent. First, it may be argued that in the context of war veterans, CBT may be less effective because the network of war memories is not sufficiently evoked or accessed, and it is possible that without special considerations and tactics in the therapy, the characteristics of war trauma and war veterans preclude sufficient emotional processing and engagement in CBT (see Foa, Riggs, Massie, & Yarczower, 1995). Furthermore, we posit that clinical trials of CBT for complex, war-related PTSD may be disappointing, in part, because the treatments evaluated are based on learning and social-cognitive models developed to account for pervasive and sustained fear and anxiety-based responses to personal life-threat or victimization (e.g., Friedman, 2006). We argue that existing CBT does not sufficiently address the needs of war veterans, because the fear conditioning and learning model (e.g., Foa & Riggs, 1995) and similar cognitive (Ehlers & Clark, 2000) and social-cognitive constructivistic models (e.g., McCann & Pearlman, 1990; Resick & Schnicke, 1993) do not sufficiently explain, predict, or address the needs of many service members and veterans who are exposed to diverse psychic injuries of war. Service members not only face life-threatening, highly fear-based trauma, but they are also exposed to horrific losses and morally injurious experiences (Nash, 2007). The grief problems that arise from traumatic loss and moral injuries have phenomenology, course, and maintaining factors that are distinct from fear-based traumas (Prigerson et al., 2009; Litz et al., 2009). Indeed, in our view, there has been a false, tacit assumption of the equipotentiality of widely varying types of traumas and traumatic contexts (Litz, 2014). For example, until recently, clinical researchers have assumed that if treatment works well with patients who have experienced civilian traumas (e.g., female rape victims), then this provides sufficient evidence that the approach as generated and tested is sufficient for deployed service members and war veterans.

We created adaptive disclosure to augment and extend existing, well-established treatments for fear-based events to target directly the complications related to moral injury and traumatic loss, as well as life-threatening trauma. In the process of developing the treatment, we considered different treatment targets and mechanisms of change, and incorporated additional intervention strategies.

ADAPTIVE DISCLOSURE

Adaptive disclosure was developed originally for active duty service members seeking care in-garrison (Steenkamp et al., 2011). We selected the term "adaptive disclosure" for two reasons. First, we wanted a name for the approach that did not employ the terms "treatment" or "therapy" because of concerns that this would deter service members who are reluctant to view their problems within a medical model. Second, the term "adaptive disclosure" captures a core goal of the therapy, namely, sharing and processing memories of war zone experiences in a therapeutic manner. In this sense, the approach is a hybrid of existing CBT strategies, specifically, a form of exposure therapy (imaginal emotional processing of a seminal event) that also incorporates some techniques used in other cognitive-based treatments (e.g., CPT), as well as techniques drawn from other traditions (e.g., Gestalt, psychodynamic therapy, mindfulness). Adaptive disclosure extends traditional cognitive and behavioral strategies by integrating them with techniques drawn from other traditions, and packaging and sequencing these techniques to address specifically the three most injurious combat and operational experiences: life-threatening trauma, traumatic loss, and experiences that produce moral injury and inner moral conflict (see Stein et al., 2012).

The therapy consists of eight 90-minute weekly sessions, which is

considerably shorter than standard CBT, in order to accommodate service members' time constraints and potential for deployment or reloca-
tion. Importantly, the treatment can be expanded as needed if duration
constraints are not relevant. The first session is used to evaluate service
member's current status, to establish the event to be targeted (the most
currently distressing, haunting, and impairing), to educate the patient
about adaptive disclosure, and to establish realistic goals. The middle
six sessions incorporate an imaginal exposure exercise whose aim is to
facilitate emotional processing of the war experience, unearth relevant
associations, and help the service member or veteran to articulate his
or her raw, uncensored beliefs about the meaning and implications of
his or her experience. If the core event is life-threat-based, these sessions are very similar to PE. However, in cases of moral injury or traumatic loss, after the basic emotional processing of the event, separate
experiential "breakout" sessions are employed. In these breakouts,
participants are encouraged to engage in imaginal conversations with
a key "relevant other" such as the deceased person being grieved or
a respected, caring, compassionate, and forgiving moral authority. In
developing the treatment, we were especially concerned that sustained
and repeated emotional processing of memories of loss or moral injury
would be counterproductive, if not harmful, if unaccompanied by
additional learning linked directly to the specific psychological injury
(e.g., shame, guilt, betrayal). Consequently, the goal of the breakout
sessions is to engender alternative emotional experiences that plant
corrective information such that the experience and internalization of
the original trauma is modified positively. Because self-condemnation
is common—especially in instances of moral injury—these imagined
dialogues offer important opportunities for perspective taking and
experiencing forgiveness. The mechanics and the flow of the middle
six sessions are depicted in the schematic in Chapter 7. The last session
is used to review experiences, underscore positive lessons learned, and
plan for the long haul in light of what was learned or at least touched
upon in the sessions.

Foundational Assumptions for Adaptive Disclosure

Adaptive disclosure is predicated on a number of core assumptions
and preconditions. First, adaptive disclosure is specifically designed
to train care providers to understand, honor, and accommodate the
military ethos, and the unique phenomenology of war trauma among
service members who may be struggling, yet preparing for their next

deployment or their military roles. We also assumed that if clinicians were knowledgeable and empathic about the military culture and were reasonably well prepared to hear about any dimension of warfare and the war experience, then service members would be more willing to build trust and feel confident that the intensively evocative and challenging disclosure and experiencing that adaptive disclosure requires are worth it.

Second, we based our approach on the premise that when treating active duty troops in garrison, the goal of the therapy should be to create a foundation for healing, repair, and recovery by presenting the treatment as an introduction of a different way of dealing with the psychological, behavioral, and spiritual legacy of combat and operational events, rather than an an endpoint. We believe that for many service members the idea of total cure or complete eradication of symptoms is unrealistic; a number should prepare themselves for lifelong challenges, especially in the context of traumatic loss or moral injury. Additionally, the complexity of the life course challenges related to exposure to war trauma, traumatic loss, and moral injuries, and the extensive treatment necessary to address these issues fully would be difficult to sustain while service members are training or otherwise preparing for future deployments.

Third, we assume that active duty service members and veterans who are new to treatment are not well-versed in sharing and disclosing their experiences. We expect that veterans' narratives will often be disorganized and unduly limited. Consequently, we assume that narratives of war zone events need to be uncovered; there is likely more to the story than the service member is willing or able to share or articulate at the start of treatment. When developing the therapy, we were mindful that disclosure and processing of shame- or guilt-based experiences would typically require more time and the development of a trusting therapeutic relationship. Yet we also knew that we did not have a lot of time to do the preparatory relationship and trust building. We assumed that honoring, respecting, and understanding the military ethos, utilizing a "no-nonsense, let's get right to it" experiential approach, and targeting issues that would resonate deeply with stress-injured service members would create a trust that would otherwise take much longer to cultivate. In this book, we provide extensive information about the military values and culture, and the multidimensional nature and sources of combat stress injuries.

Fourth, ultimately, *meaning making* is an essential change agent in all forms of psychotherapy. We were therefore especially keen to employ strategies to help service members *uncover* and clarify the *unfolding* meaning they ascribe to the experiences that haunt them. Perhaps because of the stoicism reinforced by military identity and training, prior to treatment, many service members have not sufficiently reflected on the meaning and implication of war zone harms, let alone articulated and shared these ideas. Consequently, in our view, service members need evocative experiential strategies to unearth constructions of the meaning and implication of war zone harms. We also strategically bring military roles and expectations into the therapy room. It is important for clinicians to know what a service member's job is, what his or her aspirations are or were, the degree of leadership responsibilities he or she has or wants, or would have wanted, and so forth. This knowledge helps clinicians conceptualize ways to help service members think about the implications of their damning and self-destructive ways of construing traumatic events, in terms of their identity and behavior as service members, future veterans, husbands or wives, and so forth.

Especially for nonmilitary clinicians and researchers, it is important to appreciate that the military culture and ethos foster an intensely moral and ethical code of conduct and, in times of war, that being violent and killing is normal, and bearing witness to violence and killing is, to a degree, prepared for and expected. Most service members are able to assimilate most of what they do and see in war because of training and preparation, the warrior culture, their roles, the exigencies of various missions, rules of engagement and other context demands, the messages and behavior of peers and leaders, and the acceptance (and recognition of sacrifices) by families and the culture at large. Nevertheless, service members and units face unanticipated moral choices and demands, and even prescribed acts of killing or violence may have an immediate or delayed but lasting negative impact. We contend that it is because service members have high moral standards that events that transgress deeply ingrained moral expectations cause so much inner turmoil (see Chapter 3).

Therapeutic Strategies in Adaptive Disclosure

We developed strategies to promote accommodation of the meaning and implication of various combat and operational experiences by facilitating "hot cognitive processing" (i.e., processing that is emotional, experiential, provocative; see Edwards, 1990; Greenberg & Safran, 1989) of injurious events. This is done through a combination of imaginal exposure and subsequent cognitive restructuring and meaning making (akin to the postexposure cognitive restructuring dialogue in PE). We assumed that service members would be less defensive and more open to alternative ways of construing their experience if they just shared, in a viscerally and emotionally vivid way, a poignant and painful deployment experience. In the Gestalt and emotion-focused therapy traditions, such "hot cognition" is assumed to trigger or reveal unexpressed or previously unavailable feelings, desires, and needs (e.g., Greenberg & Safran, 1989). It fosters thinking that is motivated, engaged, and focused. In a hot cognitive frame of mind, individuals are less motivated to analyze critically and their self-reflections are more raw, accessible, and immediate. This approach also helps to circumvent the defensiveness that may arise when service members are asked to think differently about a situation or event by a caregiver who does not share their experience or background. Finally, we also assumed that repeated exposure to memories of traumatic loss, acts of perpetration, or betrayal experiences without a strategic therapeutic frame for creating corrective appraisals and experiences would be counterproductive at best and even potentially harmful. Our viewpoint is that the most efficient use of time in between sessions is to foster reparation, reengagement, reconnection, and consolidation of positive meanings and improved self-care. Homework is assigned to focus on these themes (and final session strategic planning).

Similar to what takes place in cognitive therapies (Ehlers & Clark, 2000; Resick & Schnicke, 1993), we assumed that we needed to get service members to increase their awareness and insight, and to modify toxic ways of making sense of their traumas, losses, and moral injuries. Consequently, after each emotional disclosure and processing experience, the therapist ensures that there is time for a dialogue about the meaning and implication of the military trauma, and takes a very active role in addressing and influencing these emerging meanings. As a point of departure from conventional cognitive approaches, adaptive disclosure does not assume that troubling interpretations or appraisals are necessarily errant or "irrational." In some instances, self-blame may not be altogether inaccurate. In these instances, the therapist may spend less time challenging the accuracy of the belief relative to conventional cognitive therapies and comparatively more time promoting more adaptive future possibilities.

It should be noted that CPT also targets traumatic loss-related beliefs. The goal in CPT is to address/remove cognitive barriers that get in the way of an otherwise normal grief process, rather than target the loss specifically as a separate injurious experience. In CPT, patients write an impact statement about what the loss means to them, focusing on meanings regarding safety, trust, power/control, esteem, and intimacy. They also write about how the death has affected their memory of the deceased. By contrast, in order to uncover and process previously inaccessible (or nonarticulable) emotional content, we employ a "hot" cognitive experiential strategy to uncover thoughts and feelings related to the loss, somewhat akin to the approach by Shear, Frank, Houch, and Reynolds (2005). The therapist guides the service member to have an imaginal conversation with his or her lost friend. The dialogue is used to promote exposure to corrective experiences, such as "hearing" the friend say he or she forgives the service member or veteran or wants them to live a good, full life, and so forth. We believe that having the patient actively consider what the deceased would have wanted for the service member, and how he or she might want his or her memory honored, may be more effective in challenging impacted grief and guilt than would direct therapeutic challenge or Socratic questioning.

Unlike traumatic fear and loss, we did not have a precedent on which to base our efforts to heal the wounds of war-related moral injury, such as betrayal by one's leader (i.e., command decisions with lethal consequences) or acts of commission or omission that result in the perpetration of unnecessary and egregious acts of violence. In our experience working with service members, these experiences are the most toxic, yet most therapists will not treat perpetration-based moral injury within a PE or CPT framework (in PE, it is formally proscribed; Foa & Meadows, 1997; but see Smith, Duax, & Rauch, 2013 and Steenkamp, Nash, Lebowitz, & Litz, 2013). If employed to target moral injury, the premise of CPT would be that there are distorted beliefs about moral violation events that cause the ensuing misery. This, however, may not be true. In the case of morally injurious combat and operational experiences, there are instances in which judgments and beliefs about the transgressions may be appropriate and accurate, *as well as* psychologically toxic and excruciating. Furthermore, attempts to attribute these actions to the "context of war," even when appropriate, may ring hollow and/or undermine a therapist's credibility to a service member steeped in a culture of personal responsibility and moral accountability. Finally, in cognitive therapy, in-session Socratic questioning and homework assignments are used to challenge automatic thoughts about guilt and shame. In the case of moral injury, the patient would be instructed to find evidence to support or refute attribution of culpability and bad character, and so forth. We would argue that this task is enormously conflict-laden and difficult in the case of serious undeniable moral transgressions and when the war trauma is colored by betrayal stemming from previously trusted others' grave moral and ethical wrongdoing. Thus, we argue that different techniques must be used to address morally injurious military events.

Comparing Adaptive Disclosure with CPT and PE with Regard to Moral Injury

CPT (Resick, Monson, & Chard, 2014) and PE (Foa, Hembree, & Roth-baum, 2007) are disseminated as prescriptive evidence-based treatments for war-related PTSD. Proponents of these two therapies have recently attempted to argue that their respective interventions treat moral injury. Because each of these therapies explicitly attempts to address traumatic loss at least to a degree, we describe in this section we describe in this section these models' approach to moral injury, as well as the limitations of these approaches.

PE and CPT manuals do not mention the construct of moral injury, and until recently, contained minimal guidance for addressing guilt, shame, and anger related to transgressions. More recent publications have elaborated on applications of and modifications to CPT and PE for these issues (see below), briefly acknowledging a need for seeking forgiveness and making amends for deliberate acts of perpetration, but they continue to emphasize cognitive restructuring techniques designed to contextualize the transgression. "Contextualizing" entails helping patients understand that their behavior or experience was a result of the circumstances (fog) of war and that culpability is an inappropriate judgment because of role and context.

CPT was originally tested on civilian assault victims and examined in two trials with Vietnam veterans. With respect to problems related to war zone transgression, CPT attempts to alleviate guilt and anger by modifying the distorted cognitions, or stuck points (presented in the patient materials as "maladaptive," "unrealistic," or "problematic") that manufacture shame and guilt. Cognitive restructuring of stuck points related to blame and diminished self-worth, along with behavioral assignments that entail giving and receiving compliments and engaging in self-care, are CPT strategies available to alleviate the consequences of transgression. The newest version of the CPT manual (Resick et al., 2014) contains brief sections on perpetration and morality, which, again, encourage therapists to contextualize the perpetration event in terms of "who he was then with what his values and behavior are now" (p. 20) and also suggests acceptance, repentance, seeking out self- or religious-forgiveness, making restitution, or community service. Betrayal-related events are targeted by strategies that focus on seeking alternative explanations, challenging overgeneralized beliefs, and granting forgiveness to the perpetrator to attain "some peace of mind" (p. 21). No guidance is provided for implementing these new techniques, nor have they been subjected to testing as part of the treatment protocol.

It appears that the CPT framework assumes that any currently distressing event that does not involve deliberate perpetration of unnecessary violence is caused by distorted thinking that needs to be reappraised. The new CPT manual suggests forgiveness and remediation for deliberate perpetration of harms (Resnick et al., 2014, p. 78), and recommends Socratic questioning about intentionality and restructuring of distorted cognitions about control for other, potentially morally injurious (the authors do not use this term) war zone experiences (pp. 20, 76, 78). In effect, CPT appears to treat troubling war zone events as either accidents, role-consistent acts, or reactions prompted by rage, fear, or helplessness, unless the person consciously intended all the specific negative outcomes and had good choices in the moment, yet behaved badly anyway. In this way, the only way for service members to reach the threshold for real culpability is that they behaved in a sociopathic manner. This is anathema to military culture, which is deeply rooted in the moral responsibility of the intentional (not accidental) carrying of lethal weapons in war zones. In other words, CPT appears to interpret the so-called contextual morality of actions taken or not taken in combat without taking into account the warrior ethos, which allows little room for accidents or behaviors motivated by untempered emotions. Indeed, moral expectations may be violated in war through many actions or failures to act that service members consider blameworthy, even though their consequences were unintended. Examples include friendly fire, a road accident at night in the dark, or a peer being killed in a moment in which his or her trusted team member was not paying close enough attention to threats. Moral emotions can be evoked by accurate appraisals of culpability even without malicious intent. For a therapist who is unfamiliar with the military culture to assume otherwise is problematic in our view.

PE also purports to relieve guilt through *contextualizing*. The PE manual states that the combination of imaginal exposure and postexposure processing "will help the client to view the trauma in context and . . . put the events in realistic perspective" (Foa et al., 2007, pp. 28–29).

More recently, Smith et al. (2013) suggested that PE is appropriate for treating guilt associated with perceived perpetration, or harm enacted "as a consequence of the trauma context" (p. 462), which can include intentional killing while enraged. The authors state that "through repetition, new learning and disconfirmation of trauma-related beliefs can be incorporated into the [fear] structure, resulting in a reduction in PTSD symptoms" (p. 464), particularly "a more realistic view of the amount of responsibility and control during the event" (p. 468). In applying PE to transgression, the therapist elicits and explores maladaptive meanings and feelings of guilt during assessment, expands the scope of the imaginal exposure to include exculpatory contextual elements (e.g., pre- or peri-event fear or anger, postevent remorse), probes for these contextual details during the imaginal exposure, and reflects back the patient's acknowledgments of the context during processing. The suggested in-session procedures are based on the assumption that repetition will lead to therapeutic insight regarding these contextual elements and do not specify whether the therapist may be more directive and targeted in restructuring rigid beliefs (Steenkamp et al., 2013). The PE techniques for eliciting benign reappraisals are "open-ended prompts, encouragement, and reflective listening," without challenging the validity of cognitions (Paul et al., 2014, p. 280). In contrast, the therapist in adaptive disclosure is more directive, if necessary, by prompting the patient to articulate meanings in the dialog with the moral authority (e.g., "What does he or she want to tell you?"). Finally, Smith et al. (2013) state that contextualizing the transgression may be enhanced by *in vivo* exposure assignments that involve seeking disconfirming evidence of negative self-beliefs through interactions with others and seeking forgiveness or making amends. However, the incorporation of strategies promoting forgiveness and making amends (Rauch, Smith, Duax, & Tuerk, 2013) has yet to be examined empirically in service members whose traumatic events include elements of perpetration, and the relationship of moral distress to fear and fear structures remains unexplained.

In both PE and CPT, attempts at contextualizing war zone transgressions might be considered moral reassurance rather than moral repair. "Moral reassurance" is a ubiquitous coping skill in society; we use it to reassure ourselves or others (e.g., "I did the best I could," "They didn't mean to hurt me," or "Look at all the things I do right"). We suggest that for some war zone transgressions, moral reassurance might provide only short-lived relief or at worst feel disingenuous to service members. This is because moral reassurance cannot negate or invalidate troubling and painful moral truths, though it can serve as a distraction. "Moral repair," by contrast, must involve acceptance of inconvenient truths, after drawing them into as objective a focus as is possible, and tolerance of painful moral emotions, so that a new context can be created for the traumatic events going forward (e.g., by making amends, asking forgiveness, or repairing moral damage symbolically). In contrast to PE and CPT, adaptive disclosure attempts to help the patient integrate the discomfort of the moral injury through experiencing forgiveness, self-compassion, and engaging in reparative behaviors. The latter appears to be a new feature of PE and CPT, which is encouraging, but these components are not technically PE or cognitive therapy, respectively (they fit into a unique behavioral activation frame, it seems), and there are no specific instructions for carrying the assignments out or using the experiences in treatment in a sustained manner. There is also no guidance on how to proceed if moral reassurance is not possible.

In summary, to the credit of CPT researchers, in the new CPT manual (Resick et al., 2014) there is some content about how intentional perpetration should be "contextualized" or "processed" but there are no explicit exercises or developed dialogue to illustrate how that might be done. Without the latter, it is doubtful that therapists will know with confidence what to do when confronted by moral injury or whether their approach is replicable based on some operationalized standard. Other content acknowledges that self-forgiveness and separation of a past act from present totality of self are valued therapeutic goals, but detailed techniques to advance such possibilities are largely lacking. Also, to the credit of PE researchers, Smith et al. (2013) started a discourse in the PE framework to address moral injury (although the clinical recommendations are for "perceived" perpetration only). The impression we have is that CPT and PE are best prepared to help service members who are haunted by "should haves" (hindsight bias), and who shoulder an excessive amount of perceived responsibility due to a known, unequivocal, noncontingent, and horrible outcome. In these cases, it is safe to assume that self-blame is the result of unwarranted and overgeneralized distortion. However, it is unclear how CPT and PE address what we consider to be the crux of moral injury among service members, namely, guilt and shame from acts of commission or omission that entail culpability from the service member's point of view given military training and the requirements of battle. By contrast, adaptive disclosure was designed to give the military culture a place in the therapy room, place validity in the voice of the service member, accept a range of culture-consistent culpability, and target damage to moral identity by focusing on moral repair.

In adaptive disclosure, we ask the morally injured patient to have a dialogue in his or her imagination with a forgiving and compassionate moral authority or, if need be, other highly salient meaningful figures (a subordinate service member, the harmed victim, etc.). In this therapist-guided conversation, patients disclose what they have done (or how they were harmed by betrayal) and what they see as the implication of such experiences (self-handicapping, self-loathing, shame, self-destruction and abnegation, externalizing behaviors, etc.). The goal is to promote new learning through corrective feedback about the appraised implications and to introduce actively the possibility of forgiveness, compassion, reparation and repair. The approach is designed to facilitate perspective taking and to shift beliefs from blameworthiness (which may be objectively true) to forgiveness and compassion (which are nonetheless possible), and in so doing to facilitate the potential for living a moral and virtuous life going forward. Homework exercises are essential to provide exposure to corrective information to reinforce this sense of goodness and to begin the process of repair by making amends. The following assumptions guide our approach to the treatment of moral injury: (1) Pain means hope. Anguish, guilt, and shame are signs of an intact conscience and self- and other-expectations about goodness, humanity, and justice; (2) goodness is reclaimable over the long haul; and (3) forgiveness (of self and others) and repair are possible regardless of the transgression.

SUMMARY

In this chapter, we have reviewed the core conceptual underpinnings and foundational assumptions of adaptive disclosure and compared it to other treatments for PTSD. As is the case with all cognitive-behavioral treatments, adaptive disclosure employs a core set of strategies and change agents that are common to CPT, and especially PE. We repurposed some of these change agents (principally real-time evocative narration of events, i.e., exposure) and generated some novel approaches to help service members and veterans start to heal from loss- and moral injury-based harms.

CHAPTER 2

Background and Evidence

The prevailing theory about why trauma is harmful is the neo-conditioning fear-systems-based biological model of uncontrollable stress. This model is doctrine in the medical model of PTSD. The essential necessary precondition is exposure to life-threatening trauma, which triggers an unconditioned "fight–flight–freeze" response, initiating activity in the hypothalamic–pituitary–adrenal axis, the locus coeruleus and noradrenergic systems, and the neurocircuitry of the fear system. This hardwired response to life threat is richly encoded in memory and conditioned to a variety of peri- and postevent stimuli. In this framework, PTSD is in effect the manifestation of traumatic Pavlovian conditioning and learning (e.g., Norrholm et al., 2011). In discreet life-threatening contexts such as motor vehicle accidents, this model is compelling and valid from a variety of perspectives. However, in the military, in a time of war (and other complex contexts), life-threatening trauma is not the only hazard that threatens resilience. Loss, and inner conflict from morally injurious experiences, such as killing or failing to prevent unethical behavior, are coequal challenges to resilience (Nash, 2007). Each of these has a different phenomenology, etiology, and course than life-threatening experiences. Consequently, each requires a different perspective on treatment, but the focus to date has been on stress and fear.

As we argued in Chapter 1, the conditioning and learning model built on the concept of high threat and fear does not sufficiently explain, predict, or address the needs of many who are exposed to the divergent and diverse psychic injuries of war (and many other traumatic contexts). Prevention and treatment efforts need to consider different mechanisms of change, targets, and intervention strategies. What would lead to more lasting mental, spiritual, biological, and social difficulties over the long haul, a personal life-threatening experience or a child's suffering, a moral or ethical transgression in a moment of blind rage, or the grotesque loss of a special and loved member of a unit?

To put these issues in context, consider this thought experiment: What might promote a service member's healing and recovery from a single life-threatening incident, such as a sniper attack, when no one was hurt? Contrast this with a service member who is plagued by witnessing the aftermath of an improvised explosive device (IED) that killed his best friend (traumatic loss). Contrast that with a service member who is haunted by an incident where he fatally acted out his rage due to a motor attack that killed his friend the day before (moral injury related to perpetration). Compare that with the experience of a service member who is angry and demoralized over betrayal by a trusted leader whose ruthless and capricious decision led to the unnecessary death of civilians. Does the fear conditioning model fit any case but the first? Is conventional imaginal exposure, or Socratic questioning designed to challenge the accuracy of the service member's beliefs, necessary and sufficient in promoting recovery and postcombat adjustment?

Loss, especially loss as a result of violence, has a phenomenology, course, and maintaining factors that are distinct from life-threat-related traumas (Prigerson et al., 2009). Complicated or prolonged grief reactions stemming from traumatic losses share some symptomatic and etiological features with PTSD but have been shown to be distinct in a number of ways that have important implications for treatment. Specifically, although avoidance is prominent in PTSD, and is central to exposure-based treatment approaches, complicated grief reactions are often characterized by seeking out reminders of the deceased and ruminative tendencies (Prigerson & Jacobs, 2001). In fact, avoidance symptoms have been found to be only modestly predictive of traumatic loss-related distress (see Lichtenthal, Cruess, & Prigerson, 2004, for an excellent review). If, as preliminary studies suggest, individuals suffering primarily from complicated grief and loss reactions are not especially avoidant, a treatment utilizing an unadulterated, conventional exposure approach may not be optimal for such individuals. Exposure is only curative to the extent that avoidant-based coping is prominent. We argue that for service members suffering from traumatic loss (in addition to or instead of PTSD), exposure-based techniques need to be augmented with techniques designed explicitly to target other variants of posttraumatic and loss-related distress.

Combat also poses unique moral and ethical challenges, some of which have been hypothesized to create lasting harm (Litz et al., 2009). "Moral injury" is a term used to describe a syndrome of shame, self-handicapping, anger, and demoralization that occurs when deeply held beliefs and expectations about moral and ethical conduct are transgressed. It is distinct from a life threat insofar as it is also not inherently fear-based; rather, during war, moral injury can arise from killing, perpetration of violence, betrayals of trust in leaders, witnessing depraved behavior, or failing to prevent serious unethical acts (Nash, 2007). Separable from life-threatening trauma and complicated grief reactions, moral injury also requires a shift in thinking about care.

Service members who go to war are confronted with ethical and moral challenges, many of which are navigated successfully because of useful rules of engagement, training, leadership, and the purposefulness and coherence that arise in cohesive units during and after various challenges. However, even in optimal operational contexts, some combat and operational experiences will inevitably transgress deeply-held schemas about the self and humanity. Transgressions can arise from individual acts of commission or omission, the behavior of others, or by bearing witness to intense human suffering or the grotesque aftermath of battle.

Service members are uniquely at risk for moral injury not just because they are exposed to, or are perpetrators of, killing and maiming, and the grotesque aftermath of battle, but also because, for the most part, military training and culture teach service members that actions they take in war are just, moral, and ethical, and that their sacrifices are noble. Consequently, any perceived transgression is arguably particularly anguishing and disruptive, because it undermines, if not destroys, a core sustaining belief system and organizing principles. This is especially the case when previously respected and trusted leaders or peers behave immorally. One might also argue that combatants' actions, especially guerilla warfare in a civilian context, have the potential to be uniquely morally injurious, because it is impossible for even intense and realistic training to prepare service members for the surreal, unparalleled, evil acts that can sometimes occur.

The consequences of moral injury mirror the reexperiencing, avoidance, and emotional numbing symptoms of PTSD (Litz et al., 2009). That is, the transgression experience is as haunting as life-threatening and loss experiences are, and it unwittingly pervades consciousness. Consequently, service members are motivated to avoid the resulting feelings of shame and to avoid reminders of the morally injurious events. In addition, like PTSD, moral injury entails severe social withdrawal, anhedonia/dysphoria, and disinterest in previously pleasurable activities. In contrast to PTSD, moral injury is expected to lead anomie, pervasive shame and guilt, reductions in trust in self- and others in terms of moral behavior (a *broken moral compass*), poor self-care, self-harming and self-handicapping behaviors, loss of faith in God (if applicable), and, in the case of betrayal-based experiences, externalizing, blaming, and aggressive acting-out behavior.

It should be emphasized that regardless of the degree of training and preparation, and despite strong battlefield rules of engagement, warfare—especially guerilla wars of insurgency (e.g., the wars in Vietnam, Afghanistan, and Iraq)—can be inherently morally challenging. For example, in 2003, 20% of soldiers and Marines surveyed endorsed responsibility for the death of a noncombatant (Hoge et al., 2004), arguably due to the ambiguity of the enemy. Furthermore, 45% of the soldiers and Marines assessed in 2006 in a field survey in Iraq felt that noncombatants should be treated with dignity and respect, and 17% of surveyed soldiers and Marines believed that noncombatants should be treated as insurgents (Mental Health Advisory Team [MHAT-IV], 2006). Also, using a similar methodology, in 2007, 31% indicated they had insulted or cursed at civilians, 5% indicated mistreating civilians, and 11% reported damaging property unnecessarily (MHAT-V, 2008). These are putative signs of both the aftermath of moral injury and potentially morally injurious acts.

We have conducted research to examine the prevalence of the three principal war harms, namely, life threat (danger), loss, and moral injury among service members seeking treatment for PTSD (Stein et al., 2012). Before administering a clinical interview to evaluate PTSD symptoms, we asked 122 active duty treatment-seeking soldiers who had deployed to Iraq or Afghanistan to share the war experience that was the most haunting and currently distressing (this event was used to index various PTSD symptoms during the interview). We then assigned these war zone *index* events to one or more of the following categories: Life Threat to Self, Life Threat to Others, Aftermath of Violence, Traumatic Loss, Moral Injury by Self, and Moral Injury by Others. We deconstructed life threat, loss, and moral injury in this more detailed fashion, because we were interested in exploring the nuances of these experiences. The results were as follows: 40% of the events entailed a life threat either to the self or others, 30% were rated as entailing traumatic loss, 35%

entailed being exposed to the grotesque aftermath of violence, and 22% were moral injuries perpetrated by the self or others. Tellingly, in this study, the best predictor of the prototypical reexperiencing symptoms of PTSD was a morally injurious perpetration event.

We wish to emphasize that the fear conditioning model has brought tremendous advances to the trauma and PTSD field in the last 20 or so years. There has been a proliferation of clinical trials of prevention strategies (see Litz & Bryant, 2009) and well-designed trials of psychotherapies for chronic PTSD (see Bradley, Greene, Russ, Dutra, & Westen, 2005; Cahill, Rothbaum, Resick, & Follette, 2009). This work has led to extraordinary accomplishments that bring science to bear in the treatment of PTSD, and much of this work informs the care of veterans of war. For example, the research forms the basis of several noteworthy consensus- and evidence-based best-practice recommendations for the treatment of PTSD, which are very useful resources for practitioners (Forbes et al., 2007, 2010; National Collaborating Centre for Mental Health, 2005), and one specifically to inform the care of service members and veterans (see Rosen et al., 2004). In addition, the Institute of Medicine (IOM, 2007) summarized the scientific evidence that substantiates various treatment modalities, commissioned by the VA. Based on the available evidence, the most robust consensus recommendation is that CBT should be considered the prescriptive, frontline evidence-based treatment for PTSD. However, unfortunately, because most of the well-designed efficacy trials target civilian motor vehicle accident or female rape victims, it is unknown whether CBT, as designed and promulgated (standardized, relatively inflexible) is sufficient to help service members in garrison, and the available clinical trials of veterans with chronic PTSD have not been impressive.

In addition, because experts in the field have often made the assumption that all traumas and traumatic contexts are basically the same (*traumatic equipotentiality*), there has not been an adequate consideration of the unique cultural and contextual elements of military trauma; the phenomenology of warriors; or the clinical issues that arise from combat and operational stressors, losses, traumas, and moral injuries. Because of this, there are significant missing elements to care models built on CBT, especially with respect to treating active duty service members. The IOM summarized the state of the evidence pertaining to the treatment of military trauma in the following way:

> In applying a rigorous approach to the assessment of evidence that meets today's standards, the committee identified significant gaps in the evidence that made it impossible to reach conclusions

establishing the efficacy of most treatment modalities. This result
was unexpected and may surprise VA and others interested in
the disorder. Important treatment decisions for most modalities
will need to be made without a strong body of evidence meeting
current standards. (IOM, 2007, p. ix)

There have been two large-scale well-designed randomized
controlled trials (RCTs) of CBT with VA patients with chronic PTSD.
Because large-scale multisite clinical trials use varied clinical settings,
employ broad inclusion criteria, so that treated patients are similar to
patients in the community, and use well-trained and supervised but
nonexpert clinicians, the findings are more generalizable to clinical
practice, and they deserve special attention. One of the studies was a
large-scale trial of group-based exposure therapy with male Vietnam
veterans with very chronic PTSD (Schnurr et al., 2003), and the other
was a trial of individual prolonged exposure therapy with women
veterans (average age = 45 years), the majority of whom had experienced sexual assault (Schnurr et al., 2007). In each trial, the CBT was
compared to a present-centered, process-oriented group or individual
therapy. The trial with male veterans was negative (the group exposure therapy was not effective), and results of the trial using women
veterans were sobering. Although immediately after the therapy ended
and at a 3-month follow-up, PTSD symptoms were somewhat lower in
the group that was treated with prolonged exposure (with effect sizes
of 0.29 and 0.24, respectively, reflecting a small advantage of exposure
over present-centered treatment), there were no differences between
the two therapies at a 6-month follow-up.

Why are the results of clinical trials of complex war-related PTSD
disappointing relative to outcome studies targeting single-incident,
adult-onset, high-threat trauma (see Steenkamp & Litz, 2013), such as
accidents (men and women) and sexual assault (women only), and what
should be taken from these disparate results? To answer this question,
it is important to examine critically the *zeitgeist* for understanding the
psychological and biological factors responsible for the etiology and
maintenance of PTSD, and the treatment needs of traumatized individuals, namely, the fear conditioning model. In one form or another,
the fear conditioning model has guided thinking about the etiology of
war-related PTSD, from Dollard and Miller's (1950) work with World
War II veterans; through the work of Lawrence Kolb (a Navy psychiatrist during World War II) and his colleagues on the conditioned emotional response in Vietnam veterans (e.g., Kolb, 1987); to the first model
of assessment and treatment based on conditioning theory (e.g., Keane,

Wolfe, & Taylor, 1987); and, currently via attempts to prescribe prolonged exposure therapy in the VA and in the U.S. military (e.g., Karlin et al., 2010; see Friedman, 2006).

In the fear conditioning model, any trauma is construed as a serious harm or threat. This event is posited to be an unconditioned stimulus (US) that reflexively elicits biological imperatives or unconditioned responses (URs) that entail peritraumatic flight, fight, or freeze behaviors, high physiological arousal, and fear. The UR is automatically paired with a variety of contiguous peritraumatic environmental and internal phenomenological cues (conditioned stimuli [CSs]), causing strong associative bonds (conditioning). When confronted with actual or memorial representations of these CSs, a conditioned response (CR) ensues, which mimics the original peri-event UR.

In the learning framework, PTSD arguably develops because of what individuals do when inevitably faced with CSs. According to the two-factor learning precept (Mowrer, 1960), a core supplementary concept in the fear conditioning model (Keane, Fairbank, Caddell, Zimering, & Bender, 1985), if individuals succumb to the strong motivation to avoid trauma-related CSs (the "first factor"), the reduction in arousal and negative affect that ensues reinforces (via operant conditioning, the "second factor") various avoidance behaviors. Consequently, in PTSD, avoidance behaviors become automatized and habitual (and hard to change). From this, it is not surprising that developed treatments have been based on conditioning theory for phobias and other anxiety disorders, namely, exposure therapies, are the predominant treatments for PTSD (Foa, Rothbaum, Riggs, & Murdock, 1991).

In exposure therapy, the goal is the extinction of CSs, so that their association with the US/UR is reduced or eliminated. The change agent is repeated and sustained exposure to CSs, without avoidance maneuvers, which can be subtle and tenacious. Modern conceptualizations of exposure therapy (in the past, the treatment was called "implosive therapy" or "flooding"; the term "prolonged exposure" is currently in vogue) underscore the need for "emotional processing" of the CSs, which are represented in memory in networks of fear-based associations (Foa & Kozak, 1986). The "fear network" is hypothesized to contain CSs, memories of the peri-event URs and constructions related to the experience, and the experience of being harmed by the event (i.e., the meaning and implication of trauma). In order to be effective, exposure therapy requires sustained exposure to all these elements and "exposure to corrective information" (experience), such as a reduction in fear and arousal (rather than escalating terror), which creates new countervailing memories (changing the fear network).

Why is exposure less effective with veterans? Pitfalls and failures in exposure therapy are said to occur because avoidance behaviors (or difficulties in the therapeutic relationship or context) interrupt sufficient memory activation and processing, thwarting exposure to corrective experience (Foa & Kozak, 1986). In the context of war veterans, CBT may be less effective because the network of war memories is not sufficiently evoked or accessed, and it may be that without special considerations and tactics in the therapy, the characteristics of war trauma and veterans of war preclude sufficient emotional processing and engagement in CBT (see Foa et al., 1995). This may be because current approaches do not provide enough latitude and guidance about uncovering underlying toxic memories or sufficient ways to push through service members' and veterans' defenses and avoidance maneuvers during the exposure. However, signs of within-session distress during exposure therapy as practiced do not necessarily lead to posttreatment improvements (e.g., see Pitman et al.'s [1996] open trial of exposure therapy with Vietnam veterans).

It is also important to point out that the most successful trials of exposure therapies entail a combination of in-therapy exposure (via imaginal recall) and *in vivo* exposure to CSs in the environment. One could argue that the results of the exposure therapy trials with motor vehicle accident and rape survivors are so impressive because extensive *in vivo* exposure is paired with imaginal therapy (riding in a car, revisiting the context in which a sexual assault occurred, etc.). These *in vivo* contexts represent opportunities for bulls-eye exposure to corrective experiences. The same cannot be said of war trauma, especially highly distal experiences (e.g., combat in Iraq). This is not an insurmountable problem, because there are environmental triggers of the network of painful war experiences, such as news reports, conversations, emotional states, anniversaries, and sounds and smells, but their lower frequency and accessibility reduce their therapeutic value (homework assignments need to have a high probability of credibility, occurrence, and success to be effective).

CLINICAL TRIAL OF ADAPTIVE DISCLOSURE IN THE MARINE CORPS

We conducted an open trial of adaptive disclosure (funded by the Navy Bureau of Medicine and Surgery). Forty-four Marines and Navy corpsmen who deployed to Iraq or Afghanistan, and were seeking treatment for PTSD, were treated with adaptive disclosure. Because we were charged with the task of developing a very brief intervention for active duty service members who might soon be deployed again, the initial variant of adaptive disclosure was a mere six sessions. The first session was designed to conduct a needs assessment, provide psychoeducation about the intervention, and identify a target event to process. The last session was devoted to summarizing insights and gains made, and promoting adaptive ways to move forward. Accordingly, the "active" portion of treatment was extraordinarily brief—four sessions devoted to processing of morally injurious or otherwise overwhelming combat experiences.

The results were positive and reported in two peer-reviewed articles (Gray et al., 2012; Steenkamp et al., 2011). Despite being exceptionally brief (i.e., only six sessions) relative to the current iteration of adaptive disclosure, treatment was associated with clinically significant reductions in PTSD, depression, and negative posttraumatic appraisals; it was also associated with increases in posttraumatic growth. Of particular interest, there was a significant, medium-size reduction on the Cognitions about Self subscale of the Posttraumatic Cognitions Inventory (PTCI; Foa et al., 1999), but no significant reduction in the Self-Blame subscale of the PTCI. This is the appropriate and expected pattern of results for an intervention designed to treat combat-related ethical transgressions in which individuals intentionally engaged at the time but later regretted, as opposed to instances of hindsight bias in which the morally injurious act was truly accidental. Stated differently, in this study, we were able to demonstrate that improvements in global perceptions of oneself now and in the future are possible even in instances where self-blame may be warranted or unamenable to change.

The effect sizes of reductions in PTSD and depression rivaled those emerging from clinical trials using conventional exposure-based approaches to treat PTSD in military populations. Though many patients still reported nontrivial distress at the end of treatment, this was not unexpected in light of the brevity of the treatment, and unfortunately it is common even among "best-practice" approaches. Importantly, adaptive disclosure was very well-accepted and tolerated by the Marines we treated. Of particular note, the most highly endorsed item on the posttreatment satisfaction measure (with a numerical rating corresponding to *Strongly agree*) was "I would recommend this intervention to other Marines." These patients' satisfaction ratings were particularly encouraging given the constraints and practical limitations of garrison life. Finally, among the Marines treated in the original open trial, roughly one-third endorsed life-threatening danger, one-third endorsed traumatic loss, and one-third endorsed moral injury. Accordingly, adaptive disclosure appears to be broadly applicable to the varied presentations of military-related trauma that clinicians routinely see in practice.

SUMMARY

In this chapter, we have summarized the unique potential harms and traumas associated with service in war zones and have reviewed the existing evidence to support currently disseminated approaches to PTSD among service members and veterans of war. Prolonged exposure and CPT are considered first-line empirically supported interventions but each has relatively weak support in veteran and military populations. For example, the effect sizes are substantially smaller relative to those in trials using these therapies with civilians with considerably less complex trauma. Also, to date, any bona fide therapy works as well as any other—in fact, therapies that do not formally target traumatic memories do as well. Rather than sticking with the status quo, we argue that in order to advance the field and, more importantly, to improve the health and welfare of deployed service members and war veterans, it is critical to assess what is unique about war and the military culture and ethos, and to generate therapies that meaningfully account for these unique contexts. We end the chapter by reviewing the evidence to support adaptive disclosure. Chapter 3 provides an overview of the military culture and ethos to help prepare clinicians to treat service members and veterans with various psychic war wounds.

Military Culture and Warrior Ethos

"Culture" may be defined as the sum of all tangible and intangible concepts, objects, and behaviors that make up a particular way of life. The term "ethos" refers more narrowly to the values and guiding ideals that unite a group of persons who share a common identity. Culture of one sort or another is inescapable; the words you are reading right now are tools of our shared culture. Although everyone participates in one or more cultures, not everyone subscribes strongly to an ethos; not everyone shares significant facets of his or her identity with a group of other, like-minded people. Members of professions invariably do, because shared values and guiding ideals serve as the "DNA" of a professional "species," allowing it to maintain a relatively stable identity from generation to generation. As members of mental health professions, we each subscribe, more or less, to a shared ethos that belongs uniquely to our professional community. It is made up of values and ideals that are indispensable to our work, such as codes of professional ethics, a respect for empiricism, and compassion for the suffering of others. As members of warrior professions (of which there are many), service members, veterans, and even military family members also subscribe, more or less, to shared values and guiding ideals that are uniquely theirs and indispensable to their way of life. Selflessness, stoicism, and an oath to protect and defend our national identity, as reflected in the Constitution, are a few components of the warrior ethos for men and women in the U.S. armed services.

One of the bedrock assumptions of adaptive disclosure as an approach to treatment is that the cultures of those we treat, most especially their values and guiding ideals, must always be appreciated and incorporated into treatments to the extent they deserve. The process of recovering from psychological trauma of any kind, in any context, often hinges on making new meaning to explain the inexplicable, to incorporate new information into identities and world views (Janoff-Bulman, 1992). How much more must this be true for psychological injuries that occur as direct consequences of the professional activities of warfighters deployed to war zones? Consider these words by Admiral Mike Mullen, former Chairman of the Joint Chiefs of Staff, speaking about the relationship between civilians and the military at a recent West Point graduation ceremony (Shanker, 2011, p. A21):

> But I fear they do not know us. I fear they do not comprehend the full weight of the burden we carry or the price we pay when we return from battle. This is important, because a people uninformed about what they are asking the military to endure is a people inevitably unable to fully grasp the scope of the responsibilities our Constitution levies upon them. . . . We must help them understand, our fellow citizens who so desperately want to help us.

The defining act of war, killing, may only ever make moral sense in terms of the values and guiding ideals of the warfighter. Otherwise, killing is murder, an act with a very dark moral heritage. The relationship service members, veterans, and family members hold, after war zone deployments, with the once-cherished values and ideals that led them into and through their traumatic experiences in the first place may serve either as powerful risk or as protective factors: as either doorways or obstacles to meaning making, self-compassion, and acceptance. Adaptive disclosure respects the primacy, for warfighters and their kin, of warrior values and guiding ideals, and it holds the process of reconciling with them to be fundamental to treatments for war-related psychological injuries.

Our goal in this chapter is not to seduce you into falling in love with the military or its way of life. Therapists cannot help restore the psychological health of service members and veterans in their care by idealizing military culture or defending it against its critics during treatment sessions. Likewise, patients are not served by therapists who preemptively draw attention to the many faults and sometimes glaring hypocrisies of military culture, no matter how naive and self-defeating they believe their patients' conceptions of the military to be. Instead, we urge a stance of neutrality as we help service members, veterans, and military family members explore their own complex relationships with the cultures that contributed to and sustain their identities, so that they come to terms in their own way with inconsistencies and discontinuities in shared value systems and practices. Only in this way can we help service members, veterans, and military family members repair the damage that war zone experiences inflict on their personal values, ideals, and conceptions of self. Empathic neutrality—listening without judgment—may be as vital for successful therapy of a service member or veteran who has suffered a war zone psychological injury as it is for successful therapy of a couple or family system. Members of a family can criticize each other, but the therapist cannot join in that criticism without inflicting harm. Just as in the treatment of families and other systems, the therapist's job is to provide a safe place for entangled love and hate, hope and disappointment, to be explored and disentangled, so that positive identifications can be strengthened and freed from the conflicts that threaten them.

THE VALUE OF MILITARY CULTURAL COMPETENCE FOR MENTAL HEALTH PROFESSIONALS

The Departments of Defense (DoD) and Veterans Affairs have jointly recognized the imperative for all health professionals who treat service members, veterans, and military families to acquire military cultural competence, and they collaboratively have launched a series of online training modules to enhance core military cultural competencies (Department of Veterans Affairs [VA], 2009). These are free of charge and can be accessed through the VA intranet or via the DoD's Center for Deployment Psychology website at *www.deploymentpsych.org/military-culture*. This training enumerates dozens of compelling reasons why mental health professionals who treat current and former members of the military should gain competencies in assessing, understanding, and treating the military cultural components of psychological problems arising from participation in military operations. What follows are five additional considerations we hope will further motivate mental health professionals to acquire military cultural competence.

Military Cultural Competence May Enhance the Therapeutic Alliance

Although seldom studied today as a predictor of cognitive-behavioral therapy (CBT) outcomes (literature searches yield more recent articles on the role of the helping relationship in *physical* therapy than in *psychological* therapy), past reviews support the claim that the nature and strength of the relationship between therapist and patient is one of the strongest predictors of outcome, regardless which explicit treatment techniques are used. For example, after reviewing more than 100 studies that included measures of outcome moderators and mediators, Lambert and Barley (2002) concluded that relationship factors common to all therapeutic approaches account for approximately 30% of observed improvement, while specific techniques account for only 15%. Empathy, warmth, and nonjudgmental acceptance in therapeutic relationships all depend, to some extent, on therapist's accurate perception and understanding of who his or her patients are as persons embedded in their social milieus. At the very least, misconstruing or minimizing the contributions of military and veteran cultures to current patient identities can pose significant obstacles to empathic communication and effective treatment.

Military Identifications Tend to Endure

The process of becoming a soldier, sailor, airman, or Marine is arguably one of the most profound and transformative life transitions in our society. To a great extent, each inductee relinquishes aspects of his or her previous personal identity in favor of a new shared identity that is earned by passing both metaphorical and literal trials of strength and character. Once accepted into the military brotherhood or sisterhood—unless one is betrayed by it—few career Marines or soldiers willingly relinquish their identification with their military peer group, even years after taking off their uniform for the last time. Of course, many service members serve on active duty for a brief period of time without accommodating their personal identities to embrace shared military values, ideals, and practices. But for many others, especially those who served in uniform for longer than one tour, identifications with a military service branch, a military occupational specialty, and military operations overseas may be more fundamental to their personal identities than their ethnic background, race, or even gender.

Meaning Making Is an Explicit Function of Military Cultures

Military leaders are trained to use their roles as mentors to help service members make sense of the challenges, hardships, and losses they endure during military operations and deployments. How well they succeed likely depends on many factors, including the mentoring skills of the leader, the level of trust invested in him or her by members of the unit, and the nature of the challenges to their beliefs and identities that unit members endure. Meaning making is an explicit function of military leadership, just as it is of religious and political leadership. Some leaders are better at meaning making than others; some service members are better than others at adopting shared cultural attitudes, beliefs, and values as means to making sense of experiences that are otherwise incomprehensible and utterly senseless. Culturally sanctioned ceremonies, traditions, and core values also serve explicit meaning-making functions. Mental health professionals may not agree with the meaning assigned by military value systems to events experienced during deployments, especially in war zones, but they can ill afford to ignore the meaning-making power of military culture, just as they may lessen their effectiveness if they ignore explicit meanings assigned to events by religion or other cultures to which their patients subscribe.

Survivors of Traumatic Experiences Often Retreat behind Self-Protective Social Barriers

Previously called the "trauma membrane" (see Martz & Lindy, 2010), the psychosocial barrier that surrounds psychologically traumatized persons reflects a contraction of their circles of trust to exclude those whose ignorance places them at greater risk to inflict harm through uninformed judgment or unempathic carelessness. Among Vietnam veterans, this exclusionary attitude was once expressed through the often-repeated bitter declaration, "You don't know, man, you weren't there!" Careless ignorance of military cultures, roles, identities, and languages is the best way for therapists to betray the fact that they, themselves, have never been "there," and probably should not be trusted inside the trauma membrane. On the other hand, the more fully therapists understand military cultures and even speak in military language, the more easily they can empathically use their own civilian life traumas, losses, and moral injuries to earn the trust of their military or veteran patients.

Military and Veteran Cultural Factors Operating Outside the Clinical Setting May Be Robust Predictors of Outcome

To the extent service member and veteran patients participate in the military cultures within which they now or in the past lived and worked, their psychological outcomes may be determined by these external sociocultural vectors, regardless of input by the therapist. In their review of the role of therapeutic relationships in treatment outcomes cited earlier, Lambert and Barley (2002) concluded that the largest contributor to outcome is not therapeutic technique (15% of variance) or even the patient–therapist relationship (30% of variance), but factors operating outside the therapy (40% of variance). For many service members and veterans, two of the most important extratherapeutic influences are family and military peer groups, not necessarily in that order.

CHECK YOUR OWN CULTURAL PREJUDICES

In order for treating professionals to be maximally open to empathically perceiving and appreciating the cultures of service members and veterans in their care, it is helpful for professionals to become aware of their own cultural biases, and their own attitudes, political leanings, and moral feelings about the military, wars, and warfighters. We all have such attitudes and biases. American culture has yet to recover from the ideological conflicts that erupted in our country during the Vietnam War, fueled by a contentious military draft and shocking television war reporting, which together made that conflict personal for many Americans. One can argue that American culture remains divided over the meaning of the U.S. Civil War, still sometimes euphemistically labeled "The War of Northern Aggression" in the South. War is an ugly and destructive business that does not reflect the personal values and identities of many liberals, to whom the value of life is a primary consideration. At the same time, maintaining peace at all costs conflicts sharply with the ideologies of conservatives who know that the world can be a dangerous place, inhabited by people who perpetually look for ways to take what they want from others, or to impose their pattern for living on others. Personal attitudes about war and fighting wars may be even more compelling for those who have been personally damaged by war, either directly as a participant or indirectly as a family member or close friend of someone who fought in war.

Apart from moral and political convictions and preconceptions that conflict with those of their patients, therapists may find that their ability to remain neutral is challenged because of even superficial differences between their own cultural backgrounds and those of their patients. We may all be hardwired to be xenophobic to some extent: to recognize instantly the many ways in which others' language, behavior, and values may differ from our own, and to feel mistrustful and even competitive because of those differences. Human history, which can be conceived of as a continuous evolution of cultures, has largely supplanted the evolution of genotypes in our species as a much faster way to acquire new adaptive capacities, generating radically new phenotypes in decades rather than millions of years (see Nash, 1998). Like genetic evolution, cultural evolution also requires both diversity and competition for survival, except that in cultural evolution, competition is not for food or mates but for followers of ideas and patterns of living. So it may be natural for therapists to feel a visceral aversion to members of cultures that differ from their own, even slightly, and to even feel tempted to criticize or devalue others' cultures. If therapists succumb to the temptation to promote their own cultural worldviews at the expense of those of their patients, they may be perceived by their patients as hostile and dangerous rather than helpful. Cultural self-awareness and vigilant self-monitoring are the keys for health care professionals' success when working across a cultural divide.

MILITARY CULTURE: EXPLICIT AND IMPLICIT

Like all enduring ways of life, military culture includes concepts, languages, rituals, and tools that have proven themselves to be useful over time, and that have been encoded into traditions that are taught from generation to generation. It may be helpful when thinking about the many elements of military culture and subcultures to organize them into those elements that are explicitly prescribed in manuals, instructions, and other publications, and those that are less clearly written down because they are, by nature, more implicit, often operating through symbols and rituals.

Because they are clearly described in many written documents, explicit elements of military culture are relatively easy to learn about, although it may take years to master them fully. Explicit elements of military culture include hierarchies, ranks, uniforms, missions, occupational specialties, and organizational structures, as well as the multitude of acronyms and other jargon of which the military seems so fond. When treating a warfighter, or even a member of a warfighter's family, there is no substitute for learning some of these explicit elements of culture as they apply to that particular patient. There is no alternative to learning one's patient's current or former rank, level of responsibility, and defined role in the military. Rapport will be facilitated if the therapist humbly admits his or her ignorance, when appropriate, and communicates a genuine willingness to learn all the code words that must be as important for the retelling of a military deployment experience as they were for living it.

In Appendix 1, we provide a primer in the most salient explicit elements of military culture. As an adjunct, we again recommend the military culture training course developed collaboratively by the VA and DoD, available online through the Center for Deployment Psychology at *www.deploymentpsych.org/military-culture.* For the remainder of this chapter, we review the elements of military culture that may be the most powerful and enduring just because they are implicit and intangible, and cannot be shed along with the uniform: the values and guiding ideals that the warrior ethos comprises.

WARRIOR ETHOS: THE RIVER THAT RUNS THROUGH IT

Viewed from a distance, the cultures of the U.S. military appear to form a highly diverse landscape comprising four distinct service branches, each with its own highly preserved traditions, identities, roles, and languages. Yet when compared to U.S. civilian culture as a whole, military subcultures are far more alike than they are different. This is because military service members and veterans share a number of fundamental characteristics that set them apart from most men and women in America—or anywhere else in the world—who have never served in uniform. If the diversity of military cultures form a broad and varied landscape, then the river that runs through that landscape is the warrior ethos, an unchanging ideal to which all members of all military services in all eras and places have aspired. Service members differ in how closely they identify with the warrior ethos during their time in uniform, although our current professional, all-volunteer military may especially attract persons who have already chosen the warrior ethos as their personal life template. Veterans and military family members hold military values and ideals to a more varying degree, but like other facets of identity that were once cherished, the warrior ethos is seldom entirely abandoned.

A number of scholarly works have been written about the warrior ethos, such as *The Code of the Warrior: Exploring Warrior Values Past and Present* by Shannon French (2004), a professor of ethics at the U.S. Naval Academy at Annapolis, and more recently *The Warrior Ethos:*

Military Culture and the War on Terror by Christopher Coker (2007). A highly readable short text on military values and guiding ideals is *The Warrior Ethos* by Stephen Pressfield (2011), a veteran Marine and author of works of military fiction long considered to be required reading for career military officers and noncommissioned officers. The values and ideals that the warrior ethos comprises may also be glimpsed in written military codes of ethics and core military values such as honor, courage, and commitment in the Navy and Marine Corps, and the seven explicit Army values of loyalty, duty, respect, selfless service, honor, integrity, and personal courage. But no written source can fully define the warrior ethos. Like other fundamental patterns for living, its roots run too deep to be easily verbalized. Since the essential features of the warrior ethos appear in every major culture around the globe, in every era since the dawn of history, it is likely that the warrior life pattern is at least partly encoded in the DNA (collective unconscious) of our species, as Jung suggested.

The following deserve consideration as fundamental components of the warrior ethos—of military values, guiding ideals, and way of life.

Dedication to Live Every Day by a Moral Code

Morality and an explicit moral code, taught and practiced on a daily basis, are not unique to warriors. To be civilized, construction of societies must be based on moral covenants that are taught from an early age, reinforced continuously, and repaired as much as possible when broken. Religion and secular law have shaped moral codes since the dawn of civilized man and continue to play key roles in their enforcement. But in any society, in any era, people differ widely in the extent to which they really internalize moral codes, rather than merely mouthing their tenets in public, without really incorporating them into their personal goals and daily practices. Moral psychologists have used the term "moral identity" to describe the merger of moral values with self systems (see Hardy & Carlo, 2011). At one end of this moral identity spectrum lie sociopaths and the undersocialized, while at the other, at least in the ideal, lie those who dedicate themselves to embody moral covenants as their champions. Unless damaged by moral injury, warriors tend to have highly developed moral identities and to seek every opportunity, on duty or off, to champion their moral values.

Since the middle ages, warriors' dedication to moral codes has been explicitly sworn in various oaths, such as the "Oath of the Round

Table" from Mallory's 15th-century *Le Morte d'Arthur*; the 11th-century *Song of Roland* from the time of Charlemagne; and the explicit teachings of *bushido* in Japan, beginning in the eighth century. Of course, no real human warrior—as opposed to a fictionalized ideal or an incarnate god—can be expected consistently to live by an expressed moral code. Warriors take an oath to try. Compare the moral dedication of the warrior to the situation of the average civilian today, who may take only one or two limited and circumscribed oaths in the course of their lives, if ever (e.g., a marriage vow or an oath to tell the truth on a witness stand in court). Unlike the marriage covenant, there is no mechanism whereby warriors can divorce themselves from their moral relationships. They are expected to endure forever, even extending beyond their own lives in the traditions of the military organization.

Dedication to Defend the Social Order

Religious professionals, such as priests and monks, also explicitly dedicate themselves to live by moral codes, and there may be significant overlap between the professions of priest and warrior—the Shaolin monks of medieval China are an example. The warrior ethos is highly spiritual at its core. One major difference between religious and military professionals, though, is that warriors always pledge themselves not only to uphold an explicit code of conduct to the best of their ability, but also to protect the social order and promote its highest development. In the United States, the Constitution arguably serves as the soul of our social order, as is evident from its preamble:

> We the People of the United States, in Order to form a more perfect Union, establish Justice, insure domestic Tranquility, provide for the common defence, promote the general Welfare, and secure the Blessings of Liberty to ourselves and our Posterity, do ordain and establish this Constitution for the United States of America.

Each of the verbs in the preamble to the Constitution, such as "establish," "insure," and "secure," requires someone to take action, when required. They are not passive.

Enlisted members of the U.S. military all take the following oath, upon their entry into military service and periodically thereafter, to serve as defenders of the Constitution:

> I, (NAME), do solemnly swear (or affirm) that I will support and defend the Constitution of the United States against all enemies,

foreign and domestic; that I will bear true faith and allegiance to the same; and that I will obey the orders of the President of the United States and the orders of the officers appointed over me, according to regulations and the Uniform Code of Military Justice. So help me God.

Selflessness

Dedicating oneself to live by a moral code and to protect the welfare of others requires a significant commitment to selflessness: to hold the welfare of others as inherently sacred and as potentially more important than one's own life and well-being. The great sacrifices service members and their families make during war—willingly, and often without complaint—are the embodiment of selflessness. There are several ironies surrounding selflessness as a central component of the warrior ethos. The first is that the sacrifices it requires are not always perceived as sacrifices by warriors, but rather as gifts they feel honored to give, because these gifts may enrich the giver far more than the receiver. Another irony of selflessness as a core warrior value is that through offering themselves for a greater good, warriors may transcend their individual natures to become part of a much greater whole, yet without completely losing their own personal identities. They become greater versions of themselves. The reward warriors receive for their selflessness is honor, something that is revered above almost all else in the military (Pressfield, 2011).

Personal Relationship with Suffering

From the moment new recruits first get off the bus in their recruit training centers, they are taught how to suffer—physically, mentally, and emotionally. Like other aspects of the warrior ethos, the degree to which suffering is a central aspect of life in the military differs slightly from service to service, and from community to community, within military services. Ideally, suffering in the military is something that is neither sadistically inflicted on others nor masochistically inflicted on oneself, but rather taken entirely in stride, as if there were little difference between suffering and not suffering. Why set up a tent for sleeping when it takes less time to dig a shallow ditch in the ground and collapse into it, or even just drape a sleeping bag over some rocks? Why build a shelter for travelers waiting in the desert at night for helicopter transportation when the only value of a shelter is protection from the suffering caused by rain and cold? In general, warriors do not enjoy suffering, but they find meaning in it, just as Viktor Frankl (1959) did as he endured unavoidable suffering in a World War II concentration camp. Of great significance to mental health treatment programs such as adaptive disclosure, warriors may be averse to seeking mental health care unless they see some greater potential good in treatment than merely relieving their own personal suffering.

Personal Relationship with Death

As a group, warriors are drawn to death. They want to experience it up close, not as an antithesis of life but as its culmination. Warriors consider the taking of life, and the witnessing of others' deaths, necessary rites of passage, literally, baptisms of fire. One common euphemism for having experienced combat death is the phrase, "see the elephant." Another is "crossing the river." All warriors want to traverse this rite of passage, not because they lust for blood, but because they know they cannot be true warriors until they have. One may speculate that warriors attempt to master death because they, like the rest of us, fear it so powerfully. By actively seeking close, personal relationships with death, warriors at least cannot be accused of running from their deepest fears, but rather embracing them. Every variation of the warrior code prohibits taking life except when required to uphold the other central tenets of the code. Perhaps the worst possible violation of the warrior ethos—one likely to leave a lasting legacy of shame—is to run from death, to avoid it, or even be briefly paralyzed in its grip. As with suffering, the personal relationship that warriors tend to have with death may have important implications to psychotherapies such as adaptive disclosure. Combat veterans may want to know what relationship their therapists have with death. Though warrior patients may not expect their therapists, themselves, to have seen the elephant or crossed the river, they may perceive a therapist's lack of a personal relationship with death as an impediment to trust that must be overcome, somehow, before communication can continue.

Joy in Fighting

It is axiomatic that everyone possesses a certain set of talents and skills; everyone has his or her personal strengths and weaknesses. Warriors are good at fighting, and like anyone who has a particular ability, they take joy in exercising it. Warriors run to a fight rather than away from it, like most of the rest of us. Exactly what makes a warrior a good fighter is an empirical question that has not yet been answered, but certainly the ability to stay calm and focused in the face of danger must be fundamental, a capacity that likely has strong genetic determinants. Emotional, mental, and physical self-control are all crucial to effective fighting, and the best warriors enter military service with great capacities for them. Even when not fighting in combat, warriors test themselves against each other in combat sports such as mixed martial arts, one of the most popular sports in the military today. One of the tragedies for warriors who have been injured by stress is that they may lose some of their ability to remain calm, focused, and self-controlled in the face of danger; hence, they lose their ability to fight effectively. This is no less a tragedy for a warrior than for a surgeon or pianist to lose their manual dexterity. Fighters are what they are, so to try to become something else means a great loss.

Pride

Shared pride, sometimes called esprit de corps, is essential to the effective functioning of warriors in military units. Pride based on real accomplishments and abilities feeds realistic self-confidence, without which difficult military missions cannot be performed. Of course, pride is a two-edged sword. It can also be a potential obstacle to living truly by a moral code, and to the selflessness, integrity, and honesty fundamental to moral behavior. The most highly esteemed warriors lived lives of pride tempered with humility, a difficult balance to maintain. Certainly, the challenge of balancing self-esteem and true humility is not unique to the military. Heinz Kohut's (1977) psychology of the self drew attention to the need all persons have for a "healthy admiration for an idealized self-object"—someone or something outside oneself that, through identification, makes one feel more admirable about oneself. For service members who embrace the warrior lifestyle, often as adolescents, military organizations and famous warriors become their admired self-objects, as does the national flag, and the pride they feel in belonging to such great institutions translates into pride in themselves. In Kohut's view, unhealthy narcissism is based on an inability to truly admire anyone or anything outside oneself, and hence be trapped in a world without real value. The first step in becoming a warrior, even for conduct-disordered kids who end up in the military as an alternative to jail, is to fall in love with a military institution, to truly admire it and those who represent it. The next step, as with all persons' psychological development, is to internalize those aspects of external things and people that make them admirable, so that the self becomes truly deserving of respect and pride, independent of those external entities. This is surely a lifelong process, perhaps especially for members of the military. To the extent a service member's positive self-regard is grounded in their identity as a fighter of wars, he or she faces a challenge when leaving the military, for whatever reason. Loss of the military identity, and the pride that accompanies it, may be grist for the therapeutic mill when treating combat-related stress illnesses such as PTSD, which may result in medical discharges from military service or accompany other physical injuries that are incompatible with continued service.

SUMMARY

The personal identities of many members of military services are defined, to some extent, by their identifications with their service branches and occupational communities within those services. These vary widely from service member to service member, veteran to veteran, and family member to family member. Warfighters' identities also reflect, to a variable extent, the enduring warrior ethos, a highly spiritual, though not religious, devotion to living by a set of core values for the good of others. Because of their traits and lifestyles, warriors may be particularly resilient in the face of fear-based trauma and at the same time be more vulnerable to the deleterious effects of violations of moral codes or the loss of cherished attachments than others who are less devoted to moral values and guiding ideals. Therapists treating service members and veterans must learn the explicit and implicit components of military cultures, in general, and the internal world of each warrior patient, in particular. And they must build bridges of trust and respect between their own worlds of those of the warriors they treat.

CHAPTER 4

Guiding Principles of Adaptive Disclosure

It seems safe to assume that anyone reading this book is deeply affected by war, personally or professionally. You may be a service member or veteran, you may care for or treat service members or veterans and want to learn new strategies, you may be a professional who wants to start treating service members or veterans with PTSD and related problems, you may have a loved one who is in the military, or you may be a concerned citizen who wants to be informed. We all come with our own assumptions and biases about the impact of war and what military personnel need to heal from the enormous and deep psychic wounds they suffer. In this chapter, we share our biases and assumptions, our treatment philosophy. It is important to appreciate the conceptual underpinnings of adaptive disclosure. This information is especially critical to guide professionals who intend to use the treatment as we prescribe it, because they might need to accommodate a change in *their* clinical assumptions. It is also important for those who pick and choose various adaptive disclosure elements, or assimilate adaptive disclosure into their own approach.

As stated at the outset, adaptive disclosure aims to help service members and veterans recover and heal from combat stress injuries and PTSD. It promotes coming to terms with the meaning and implication of the three core types of traumatic war experiences (life threat, loss, moral injury) and reducing toxic or damaging ways of construing their long-term impact. For many, this is a lifelong challenge that is dependent on personal resources, one's family, the community, the culture, the health care systems, and government (e.g., financial compensation for service-connected problems). How much weight should we put on individual psychotherapies, and more to the point, how much should healing and recovery depend on adaptive disclosure specifically?

LENGTH OF ADAPTIVE DISCLOSURE

Adaptive disclosure was designed originally to be a brief therapy (six sessions). We took this tack for two reasons. First, our original work was with service members with considerable time (and patience) constraints. Second, unlike the current *zeitgeist* among evidence-based therapies, we assume that any psychotherapy is a starting place rather than a prescriptive dose of a treatment that cures (or does not). Examination of mean symptom levels at "posttreatment" in even the most compelling treatment–outcome studies confirms that, with most patients, there is more work to be done. Third, we assume that lasting change can come only from real-life and extratherapy exposures to corrective experience. In other words, individual psychotherapy is never sufficient to produce lasting healing from serious war trauma. If a given service member or veteran only develops an intimate and trusting therapeutic relationship with his or her therapist and only uses the therapy hour to try out various new ways of feeling safe, or to grieve, or to find forgiveness, he or she will not change in lasting and meaningful ways. Consequently, we designed adaptive disclosure to be a vehicle to plant healing seeds and to set a process of lifelong healing and recovery in motion. Even if patients have benefited terrifically from the therapy in diverse ways and they no longer have PTSD, we use caution and help them plan for potential relapses and tough periods ahead, especially in the case of severe guilt from traumatic loss and various moral injuries.

If these assumptions are valid, how many sessions are required to start a healing process? We recommend adhering to the eight-session approach described in this book. Yet there were ample times during our research piloting and testing of adaptive disclosure that therapists (and supervisors) and patients were frustrated with the brevity of the treatment. More processing sessions are to be expected in complex cases and should be negotiated collaboratively with patients. But we urge therapists to use adaptive disclosure as designed, namely, to initiate a process and plant useful seeds for a different way of coping with combat stress injuries over the long haul, and not as a total alleviation of conflict and suffering.

GOALS FOR ADAPTIVE DISCLOSURE

Although we offer adaptive disclosure as a means of planting healing seeds for the future, it is nevertheless essential to be hopeful that positive and lasting change is possible. In broad terms, therapists should expect that by providing service members and veterans with a compelling, meaningful, and useful encounter with difficult principally harming experiences, adaptive disclosure can teach them that: (1) Approaching psychologically painful material is a viable alternative, and feared consequences from doing so (e.g., losing complete control or being entirely overwhelmed) do not occur; (2) processing and reconsideration are useful ways of seeing that certain deployment experiences can change (patients can examine, monitor, and accept—rather than be defined by—what they did, what they saw, what others did, how someone was lost, etc.); (3) shameful or guilt-inducing material can be shared without permanent diminishment or rejection; (4) vulnerability can be tolerated and successfully navigated; and (5) patients can reclaim good parts of themselves that they have lost since deployment (e.g., reconnecting with previously valued and enjoyed activities and people).

PTSD is characterized by a downward spiral of compounding events. The initial traumatic event leads to emotional and physical dysregulation, and a fear of being overwhelmed by terrible thoughts and feelings. It also leads to maladaptive changes in beliefs (schemas) about the self and world. The effort to avoid reminders of the event (triggers), and the consequences of changes in important schemas, pulls people away from positive and reparative encounters with others and into subtle and overt patterns of isolation and self-harm. This, in turn, leads to more psychological impairment and life injury. However, just as there are spirals of harm, spirals of healing are also possible, in which mastery and engagement lead to more efforts at mastery and more contact with others. These experiences, in turn, nourish and enhance one's life by providing reparative experiences. Adaptive disclosure is intended to facilitate a healthier spiral of response. By providing a positive experience of approaching extremely difficult material in the presence of another person, it is hoped that, over time, the experience will become a reference point for what is possible and desirable, and as a function of this, will facilitate increased help seeking, processing, and engagement with others.

The goal in every case is to begin to repair, reclaim, recover, and rehabilitate. It is particularly important to facilitate approaching and utilizing resources for healing *within the person's world* (e.g., the military), in the form of connections with peers, leaders, family members, physical training, and so forth. Memory is a constructive process. Each time a memory is taken out of storage, it is modified. Therefore, other relevant information, new interpretations of the experience and what it can mean, as well as the response of the therapist to the disclosure, will become attached to the initial memory, modifying the patient's subjective experience of it. In adaptive disclosure, exposure is used both to facilitate more complete processing of a representative traumatic event (typically one among many), and, equally importantly, help the patient be as receptive as possible to new, more adaptive interpretations of the trauma. Using exposure, the therapist promotes an emotionally intense engagement with painful military experiences. It is assumed that this kind of engagement will render the "psychic soil" receptive and facilitate hot cognitive processing of alternative, more adaptive constructions of the experience (as opposed to passive, unemotional, and strictly intellectual dialogue).

The proximal and most important aim of adaptive disclosure is to promote accommodation and adaptive meaning making of the worst or most pressing combat and operational trauma or experience. This is accomplished by first implementing an *exposure component*, which entails asking service members to relive—through vivid imagination—a salient combat and operational event. During, and especially after, the service member shares various visceral experiences and thoughts, the therapist directs a dialogue that promotes adaptive meaning making and perspective taking about the implication of the experience for the service member moving forward in his or her life. The intent of adaptive disclosure, then, in contrast to conventional approaches, is not just to demonstrate that memories and their accompanying emotions are tolerable or that interpretations are irrational, but that there are more adaptive possibilities as one moves forward. The haunting combat experience need not be destiny; it need not forever define the service member. Service members also engage in homework exercises designed to continue to expand corrective processes outside of session. If the focal experience is a life threat, then exposure and the meaning-making dialogue is used exclusively. However, if the salient event is a *combat and operational loss*, the therapist follows the exposure component with a perspective-taking exercise, asking the service member to have a conversation with the lost comrade. If the experience involves a moral injury, the exposure component is followed by a different perspective-taking approach, in which the service member is asked to have a conversation with a compassionate, forgiving, and benevolent moral authority, someone to whom he or she would be a mentor, or perhaps the actual victim (in perpetration cases)/perpetrator (in betrayal cases).

A THERAPIST'S STYLE AND STANCE

Adaptive disclosure requires a *directive* stance and approach. Therapists need to be participant–observers, with heavy emphasis on participation. They need to be keenly engaged and, when needed, to behave like a director who is also an actor by trade, assisting another actor struggling with a part in a stage play. Indeed, adaptive disclosure encourages patients to be *method actors* to a degree. Engaging a patient at that level requires training, modeling, practice, and coaching. In adaptive disclosure, we ask patients to attempt not only sharing and reliving of emotional memories (or experiencing them for first time) but, in the case of loss and moral injury trauma, also to literally take on the role of or imagine the perspective of their dead friend or a forgiving and compassionate moral authority in real time and in the first person. This can be tremendously challenging for most. It requires a therapist to have not only great compassion and humility but also to provide guidance, direction, and at times, to chime in evocatively and sometimes even provocatively in assuming the role of these compassionate actors.

One of the reasons we have emphasized the importance of knowledge about the military culture and ethos, and understanding of what is harmful during and after battle, is that adaptive disclosure therapists need to infer ideas about what is not being expressed by patients: What do patients need to say and feel but are unable or reluctant to do so? The reason for this is that with respect to loss and moral injury, in this therapy, we need patients to articulate in an evocative emotional way what people who know and love them would say about the reasons they give for their own self-condemnation, guilt, and shame. This is a serious responsibility. Even in the best of circumstances, we urge therapists to be unassuming and to treat their inferences *as hypotheses* and test them by their impact on the process. For those professionals who do not have experience being directive and actively engaged in an evocative manner, this will require practice and perseverance.

The therapeutic stance needs to be a direct, trustworthy, warm, and fully engaged one. Very importantly, it should be respectful and collaborative. Both the therapist and the service member/veteran bring essential expertise to the work at hand. Therapists know about the lasting impact of trauma and about stress and coping, and patients are experts in their culture and their own experiences. Both domains of knowledge are critical for the work to be successful. This approach differs from supportive and analytic perspectives in that it is more directive and assertive; it differs from traditional exposure treatments in that it specifically acknowledges and targets aspects of posttraumatic suffering other than fear and anxiety (e.g., guilt, shame, moral failure, grief, changes in identity, and expectations). This approach rests on the assumption that the service member or veteran already has the resources he or she needs to do this work; we are simply helping him or her to access these resources in a new way. Finally, all of the work needs to be informed by an awareness of military ethos and values, as well as an understanding of the phenomenology of combat.

The goal is to listen to determine what anchors the experience as an insurmountable problem. In addition to the primary themes of fear, grief and loss, and moral injury, examples include fear of loss of control; severe conflict; unmitigated self-reproach and/or reproach of others; and fear of regression to a less competent self.

In all dialogues, the therapist needs to listen for catastrophic expectations and actively generate hypotheses about what is experienced as insurmountable. Direct questioning should be used to help formulate a working understanding of core sources of suffering, and these should be reflected back to the service member or veteran for his or her evaluation and elaboration. Any inference needs to ring true for the service member or veteran. Within any trauma, there will be many themes (i.e., issues, implications, meanings, ways of interpreting experience), but some themes are more unapproachable than others—these are the themes for which to listen. Often, clues to the most deeply troubling themes can be assessed in formal ways with paper-and-pencil questionnaires or described through the service member's narrative. It is worth also listening for what is not said, what is likely to be shame-laden and reflect poorly on the self, and themes that drive important changes in identity and characteristic ways of relating to other people. Because patients may be more hesitant to bring up these experiences, the therapist initially may need to be the one to address them in a Socratic manner. In general, it is useful to think about the possible symbolic or functional meaning of symptoms and dysfunction. For example, a service member may describe a terrifying event in which fear is certainly salient, but the issue that causes him to cringe away from his life may be less the fact that he was deeply frightened or threatened, and more that the fear caused him to hesitate, thereby dishonoring himself or endangering comrades. Thus, the exposure might begin with the fear-based recollection but move quickly on to the implications for his schemas about himself and his worth.

It is typically best if new perspectives feel as though they emerge directly from the service member or veteran. The exercises that target loss and moral injury in adaptive disclosure can facilitate this. Other options include referencing the types of experiences and understandings other patients have had, mapping one's language onto the patient's whenever appropriate, and staying as close as possible to the patient's frame of reference while still bringing new perspectives to bear.

One of the advantages of an experiential approach to trauma treatment is that it relies less on what patients have verbal access to when asked various probing questions and relies more on unfolding real-time emotional reactions. In addition, when exposure is successful, it leaves the service member or veteran more receptive to the therapist's input. This receptivity is a form of suggestibility. Making therapeutic use of suggestibility requires attention to language. All language should affirm the idea that the needed resources (including the capacity to access and utilize help) lie within the individual, that positive change is possible and will evolve over time, and that the impact of one's deployment experiences need not be fixed. In addition, it is advisable to avoid leading with a negative statement ("You can never leave these experiences behind") and instead emphasize the positive, even when it requires modification ("You have it in you to grapple with these painful experiences in ways that will lead to positive changes over time, and while everyone is affected by combat, you are learning ways to engage these experiences that are more adaptive and lead to greater wisdom and perspective, which will serve you going forward").

THE NEED TO DIG DEEPER

Finally, another principle of adaptive disclosure that distinguishes it from CBT approaches to PTSD is that we assume that, in most cases, service members and veterans need the right context to uncover memories and constructions of their traumatic experience(s). It is not that we assume some memories or specific aspects of a memory are repressed because of some putative unconscious motivation. Rather, we assume that some aspects of a traumatic experience may be unwittingly inaccessible, and therapists should be ready for newly accessed and consequently formative memories. Therapists need to assume that because most service members and veterans have done incomplete remembering and processing of their trauma at best, what they understand and have been told at the outset is not necessarily what they get. The assumption is that the level of emotional activation and engagement may lead the patient to uncover or disclose deeper, more problematic issues as the exposure and experiential exercises proceed. The uncovering might come in the form of a modification of the salient aspects of a trauma or the key conflictual elements of an experience. Some patients reveal a new memory that they knew from the start was the most troubling experience but were unable to disclose because of shame (e.g., a personal transgression). Needless to say, this underscores the importance of being nonjudgmental, nonmoralistic, caring, compassionate, and understanding.

SUMMARY

In this chapter, we have provided detailed information about the goals for adaptive disclosure, and the therapeutic style and process that provides the backbone for specific change agents and techniques. We underscore the need for clinicians to be nonjudgmental, nonmoralistic, open to accepting the lived experience of service members and veterans, and open to the need to dig deeper and uncover unacknowledged or shared memories.

CHAPTER 5

Assessment, Case Conceptualization, and Treatment Planning

One of the attractive aspects of systematic manualized cognitive-behavioral approaches to treatment is that each patient's treatment is evidence-based; each case is a single-case clinical trial. In adaptive disclosure, it is important for clinicians to establish baseline using a psychometrically sound structured diagnostic instrument (we recommend the Clinician-Administered PTSD Scale [CAPS; *www.ncptsd. va.gov*]). One question that needs to be answered is does this patient have PTSD; that is, is PTSD the right primary and guiding clinical schema to use for the patient at this time? A PTSD diagnosis is not strictly an issue about the validity of the label in terms of how to best conduct and focus care (and to determine whether formal mental health care is the right path). The label also carries a highly significant meaning for service members, peers, leaders, family members, and employers, and it has implications for financial compensation for service-connected disability.

The other question that needs to be addressed is how this patient is doing each week; is he or she getting better? This is accomplished by weekly administrations of a paper-and-pencil questionnaire, such as the PTSD Checklist (PCL; Weathers, Litz, Herman, Huska, & Keane, 1993). Monitoring change is a win–win situation. For example, patients learn to be better consumers of treatment (e.g., "Am I getting what I need?"). Also, self-monitoring of PTSD symptoms has been shown to promote change. This is for good reason. Self-monitoring and symptom tracking help the patient realize that symptoms fluctuate for systematic reasons (e.g., a stressful week or exposure to reminders). An understanding of the link between internal and external events and PTSD symptoms can also reduce confusion and help patients to focus their attention on working strategically to plan, manage, and cope with various provocations rather than to avoid them altogether, which never works. Monitoring also allows clinicians to discern whether their efforts and the tack taken at any given point in therapy have been fruitful, or whether the approach needs to be modified in subsequent sessions.

Because most service members and veterans seeking treatment for war-related PTSD have complicated and interrelated biological, mental, social, spiritual, and behavioral problems, the initial assessment should also be used to conceptualize each case especially in terms of the extent to which various problems are trauma-linked. In other words, when a patient has many problems, all of which may be legitimate separate targets for treatment, to what extent are various problems posttraumatic? Adaptive disclosure should be considered a first option when it can be reasonably expected that there would be positive collateral change when a focal trauma and its meaning and implications are processed. Even if this is the case, it is still prudent to generate a treatment plan and prioritize targets for intervention (e.g., a crisis may need to be addressed, or a pressing non-deployment-related mental health problem requires attention). In preparation for adaptive disclosure, additional goals entail (1) determining whether the therapy is appropriate given the patient's current resources and capabilities (e.g., is a high-demand, emotionally intense therapy indicated at the present time?); (2) establishing the principal war-related harm that is most pressing on the patient's mind and the most currently distressing; (3) creating a working conceptualization of ideographic themes that will need to be processes during the therapy; (4) assessing buy-in about the therapy (once explained); and (5) redressing obstacles to compliance and engagement.

The following are necessary assessment tasks and specific questions that can be asked to gather necessary information:

ASSESS CURRENT FUNCTIONING

"OK, then, can you please tell me how you have been doing lately?" The therapist should listen for symptoms of PTSD, other mental health problems, and problems in functioning (if the patient is a service member, within and outside the military). The therapist should also listen for problems that may get in the way of compliance with care (i.e., prognostic of likely no-shows). These obstacles need to be addressed head-on collaboratively.

ASSESS DESIRED CHANGE

"Of all of the problems we just discussed, what would you like to see change most? How would you like things to be different? What kind of help do you think you need (what might be most helpful)?" These questions are designed to evaluate the degree to which the patient is hopeful but realistic about changes he or she would like to happen. The therapist will need to know whether the patient has a particularly bleak/pessimistic outlook or—equally problematic—a naively optimistic expectation for therapy. Throughout adaptive disclosure, it will be necessary for the therapist to instill hope while tempering unrealistically high expectations (e.g., the complete elimination of combat-related distress/impact is an unrealistic expectation). Hopeful expectations can and should be cultivated, provided that the hope centers on developing a viable and fruitful path forward as opposed to eradicating all distress by the end of formal treatment.

If the patient is particularly pessimistic, the therapist needs to identify this expectation as being part of the problem itself, in other words, part of the posttrauma condition in which trauma casts a shadow over the present and the future, thereby unduly diminishing optimism. The therapist should go on to suggest that the treatment will diminish this pessimism. By processing combat experiences and reengaging with seemingly lost aspects of self, the shadow of postdeployment darkness should begin to lift and allow the process of recovering from combat begin. The patient is not being asked to adopt a superficial optimism but rather to identify some of his or her pessimism as linked to personal experiences, and to at least consider the possibility that the work of the next few weeks may result in a change in expectations about the future.

If the patient is expecting a dramatic shift in functioning, the therapist will need to be realistic about the pace of recovery from combat and operational stress injuries. Without dashing hopes, it will be important to not only to validate those aspirations, to suggest that the intervention is designed to jump-start that process, but to also note that there are no quick fixes given the magnitude of change resulting from combat. State that the intervention is designed to be brief and is intended as an example of how change can occur moving forward over the long haul. Furthermore, it is helpful to explain that significant change happens slowly through an action–reaction process in which healthier behaviors and thinking patterns are rewarded, creating better adaptation over time. In other words, the therapist may express confidence in the ultimate goals envisioned by the service member, while simultaneously explaining the limited duration of the intervention and the gradual nature of recovery from combat stress.

In addition to gathering information about what is causing the patient to suffer, these questions give the therapist a sense of the patient's verbal facility, the degree to which he or she is aware of the problems, how he or she thinks about what has happened and why, and whether he or she can articulate what he or she hopes will change. Some patients might provide only short, terse, and poorly articulated accounts. If that happens, this is a clue about how things might go in the therapy, and it might mean that the therapist will have to be more directive and ask questions to uncover tacit content, or content that the patient has not yet thought of.

ASSESS PREDEPLOYMENT FUNCTIONING

Ask questions such as "Tell me a little bit about why you joined the military"; "What were you like before you (first) deployed?"; and "I want to get a sense of how you started out." Knowing why the service member joined can be very helpful. Listen for idealistic notions he or she had about the military prior to joining, beliefs about wanting to help others, feeling as if it was his or her responsibility to do so, wanting to get away from family problems, or simply wanting the excitement of killing others. This will help the therapist to conceptualize who the patient is as a person and ways in which his or her expectations may have been violated by actual experiences during war. Ask the patient to share how he was as a service member and as a person. Listen for themes of goodness, confidence, energy and commitment, engagement with others, good friendship, hopefulness, positive self-regard, faith in the goodness and trustworthiness of authority figures (and other people in general), and belief in fairness and the inevitability of justice. Over the course of the therapy, these schemas will need to be contrasted with how the patient is now. It may be difficult for patients to recall what they were like before deploying, particularly if they have had multiple deployments or are (were) career service members and have been in the military for a long period of time. The therapist may want to ask about what patients were like either before joining the military, or before their first deployment. It also may be helpful to ask them how others (e.g., a family member or spouse) would have described them prior to deployment.

ASSESS THE PRINCIPAL HARM

If therapists use a structured clinical interview to establish PTSD and the severity of specific PTSD symptoms, the event used for contextual questions about various symptoms (called the "index trauma" or "event") is the war experience that currently is the most distressing. The index event generated for this purpose in most cases will be the principal harming event targeted (initially) in adaptive disclosure. However, if there is concern that there might be another event, or if therapists prefer to use a dialogue to generate discussion of the principal harm, he or she might say the following:

> "I want to get a sense of what aspects of your experiences in Iraq [or Afghanistan] are bothering you the most and are making it hard to move forward. One way to approach this is to choose an event that is most haunting you or is currently the most distressing. I understand that it may be hard to select one event out of many. However, I suspect there are a few that stand out more than others. Usually it is one that keeps coming back to you in nightmares or keeps popping into your head throughout the day when you don't want it to. Can you think of an event during your deployment that you've had a really hard time getting over? I don't need to know all the details at this time. If you are willing, would you spend a few minutes briefly describing this experience?"

Allow some time for the service member or veteran mentally to generate a few possible difficult experiences that might be the focus of the intervention in coming weeks. Tell him or her to take a couple of minutes to think about recurring memories that have been particularly stressful. If he or she is unsure about whether an event/memory is appropriate, you can offer examples (seeing someone die or be hurt, doing or not doing something one feels he or she should have done/not done), or you can suggest that the service member run the events he or she is thinking of by you for your input.

If a number of possible target events emerge, it may be useful to develop a hierarchy by having the service member use a 10-point rating scale. Have the patient choose a few different incidents that are bothering him or her and while briefly discussing each one have the service member rate them on a scale from 1 to 10. Specifically, an event that would be rated as a "1" would not be distressing or upsetting in the slightest and an event that would be rated as a "10" would be the most distressing/upsetting experience he or she can conjure up. If the patient believes the most distressing (i.e., "10") experience will be difficult but manageable, then it may be an appropriate index event to use for subsequent exposure sessions. It is important to be very clear, however, that a helpful/successful intervention does not require this. As long as an event is selected that is at least moderately distressing (i.e., > "6"), it will likely be a beneficial experience. It is better for the patient to experience mastery of an experience that is a moderately distressing event during exposure than to attempt to process an inordinately distressing event in six sessions and make little progress.

Once the service member or veteran has identified a traumatic event, spend some time discussing why he or she has chosen this event as the worst (or one of the worst) event, so as to assess whether this is truly a difficult issue for him or her.

ASSESS HOW THE PATIENT IS NOW (ESPECIALLY AS REFERENCED BY THE LEGACY OF THE PRINCIPAL HARM)

"What are you like since this experience happened to you? What's different?" Particular changes to inquire about, and to be sensitive to, include (1) self-opinion, (2) hopefulness and optimism, (3) relationships, (4) trust in others and trust in oneself, (5) perceptions of control and competence, (6) optimism about life in general, and (7) feelings of safety. Look for and acknowledge positive changes (e.g., maturity and growth), as well as changes that interfere with life performance (as a service member or in other roles), well-being, and quality of life.

The goal is to listen for whatever anchors the principal trauma experience as an insurmountable problem. In this dialogue, the therapist needs to listen for catastrophic expectations. In addition to the primary themes of fear, grief and loss, and moral injury, examples include (1) fear of loss of control, (2) severe conflict, (3) unmitigated self-reproach and/or reproach of others, and (4) fear of regression to a less competent self. Hypotheses as to what is experienced as insurmountable should be examined through direct questioning. Any formulation the therapist makes should be reflected back to the service member or veteran for his or her evaluation and elaboration. It needs to ring true for the service member or veteran. Furthermore, the therapist should assume that there is a reasonable likelihood that the central target will shift over the exposure sessions. Although the time is brief, the level of emotional activation and engagement may lead the service member or veteran to uncover or disclose deeper, more problematic issues as the exposure proceeds. The therapist should be prepared to adjust his or her therapeutic focus accordingly.

Within any trauma, there will be many themes (i.e., issues, implications, meanings, ways of interpreting experience), but some themes are deemed by the patient to be more unapproachable than others—these are the themes for which to listen. It is also worth listening for what is not said, what is likely to be shame-laden and reflect poorly on the self; these themes drive important changes in identity and characteristic ways of relating to other people. As patients may be more hesitant to bring up these experiences, the therapist may initially need to be the one to address them in a Socratic manner. In general, it will be useful to think about the possible symbolic or functional meaning of symptoms and dysfunction. For example, a service member or veteran may describe a terrifying event in which fear is certainly salient, but the issue that causes the service member to cringe away from his or her life may be less the fact that he or she was deeply frightened or threatened, and more that the fear caused him or her to hesitate, thereby dishonoring himself or endangering comrades. Thus, the exposure might begin with the fear-based recollection but move quickly on to the implications for the service member's schemas about him- or herself and self-worth.

WRAPPING UP THE ASSESSMENT AND PREPARING THE PATIENT FOR ADAPTIVE DISCLOSURE

Not unlike other focused, short-term approaches to PTSD treatment, adaptive disclosure requires that patients be ready to get to work and willing to commit and focus on processing traumatic experiences. A well-suited patient is one who is not dealing with other pressing stressors and adversities that may interfere with or distract from engagement in the therapy. Patients also need to be able to tolerate negative affect and the possibility of feeling more pain before feeling better, and to understand that the therapy is a start, not a finish. Service members and veterans should be motivated to suffer less or to be less impaired in their work or home life and therefore willing to entertain personal change. Patients who are particularly self-condemning or angry about mistreatment and betrayal may have extremely tenacious beliefs, so, in these instances, seeking therapy should be seen as a sufficient tacit sign that some part of the person thinks there might be a different way forward. In any event, patients should, at least, be open to the idea that there are things that they can learn to alter their path.

The therapist should wrap up the assessment by summing up what has been learned and asking the patient whether what he or she is hearing feels right. Any feedback and recommendations should be followed by sufficient time for the patient to ask questions and to express concerns about what is going to happen over the course of the therapy. It is vital that the therapist gets feedback about whether adaptive disclosure is something that the patient would like to try. We recommend that a verbal "contract for care" be established, with clear expectations for therapist and patient.

What should be avoided is producing an inadvertent failure experience brought on by the patient's problems tolerating the treatment or poor compliance and engagement. We do not want to confirm patients' expectations that they are incapable or hopeless. We also do not want to waste patients' time with the wrong type of approach or provide false expectations about relief that may not be forthcoming. Any reluctance should be taken seriously and discussed in detail. If therapist and patient determine that adaptive Disclosure is not appropriate, it might be useful to discuss a contingency plan. That is, what would be signs that the approach would be indicated? Then, if the therapist does some other type of therapy with the patient or supportive work, a reassessment of appropriateness would be expected by the patient, and he or she could take co-ownership of monitoring his or her status and deciding about whether to start adaptive disclosure. If the therapist judges that a reticent patient is appropriate for adaptive disclosure, he or she should consider inviting the patient to try the approach and be especially attentive to getting the patient's feedback about how each session goes (e.g., were his or her concerns realized?). In the planning and summing up dialogue, the therapist might say:

> "Sometimes it takes time and focus to really appreciate what has changed for you. Combat changes everyone, but it is possible to make choices about what that change looks like. You need to do this before you can generate a plan of action to become who you

want to be. This includes reclaiming some of who you were before, as well as keeping the best of what you have learned from being a service member and being in combat. My goal is to help you do that. I want you to learn that you can reclaim and begin to reestablish the good parts. But first we have to get clear on the differences between now and then."

SUMMARY

In this chapter, we have reviewed assessment strategies that will help clinicians and patients prepare for adaptive disclosure. Clinicians are well advised to conduct a formal structured clinical evaluation of the PTSD symptom burden. This process requires the identification of a principal harm (otherwise known as an "index event"), which is required to individualize adaptive disclosure. We have shown that index events can be categorized into life threats, losses, or morally injurious experiences (Stein et al., 2012). We also have provided a set of questions designed to help the clinician appreciate who the service member or veteran was before the exposure to war trauma, how he or she is now (which may be many years after discharge from the military), and to discuss how the service member or veteran would like use the therapy to change.

CHAPTER 6

Beginning Adaptive Disclosure

Session 1

This chapter describes what therapists need to do and what they should tell patients in the first formal session of adaptive disclosure. This first session should be preceded by at least one formal assessment session (see Chapter 5). If the patient is judged to be appropriate for this therapy, therapists should start the session providing feedback about diagnosis and the initial case conceptualization. This should cover the idea and import of tackling a principal harm even if there are multiple war traumas. The rest of the first session is devoted to introducing and describing the therapy, getting patient feedback and buy-in, and setting the patient up for his or her first exposure session (which will be Session 2). The first session might be covered in an hour. However, subsequent adaptive disclosure sessions require up to 90 minutes. In the following chapters that depict actual therapy instructions, we provide specific standard narrative (*in italics*) that should be used as a guide for not only what needs to be covered but also how it should be covered. The main foci of each session are depicted with italicized sample dialogue, but this sample should not be taken as a script to read. Rather, therapists can adapt it to the needs of the patient and to suit their own professional styles.

INTRODUCING ADAPTIVE DISCLOSURE (WHAT IS IT?)

The keys to impart about adaptive disclosure are (1) what the label means and implies; (2) that the therapy was designed specifically to help service members and veterans; (3) that retelling in imagination is a core strategy; (4) that retelling is necessary but not sufficient, and depending on the principal harm or initial focus of the therapy, additional imaginal dialogues with "relevant others" may be necessary; (5) that in-session experiences need to be augmented by homework and, ultimately; (6) lasting change requires reengagement, reattachment, forgiveness, and self-care; and (7) that the therapy is intended to start the process of healing—the scars of war are deep, so the therapist and patient need to work together to think of a long-haul pathway and plan to continue the positive lessons learned in the therapy (and to counteract any tendencies that arise to take steps back). Here's what to cover in introducing adaptive disclosure:

> "I recommend that we start a treatment called adaptive disclosure. The therapy has this name because it is believed that it is helpful to talk about (or 'disclose') difficult events in order to move past them—you have to look back so you can look forward. This doesn't mean 'spilling your guts' to everyone you meet, but rather you are learning to talk about what has happened in a useful way. The goal is not necessarily to take away all of the problems you are experiencing, but rather to provide you with an example of how coping with your experiences can look different to you when you talk about them rather than avoid them. Part of what we'll do is to help you figure out what 'adaptive disclosure' is for you: who you share your experience with, how much you choose to share, and when you decide to share it. By talking about some of the more difficult things that happened when you were deployed, rather than just pushing them away or avoiding them, you can sort through them and move forward."

DESCRIBING THE MAIN GOALS OF ADAPTIVE DISCLOSURE

Once you have introduced adaptive disclosure, highlight specific goals of the therapy, to give the patient a sense of the work that will be involved:

"In a way, combat and operational stress injuries are like physical injuries: They need the right diagnosis, so that the right treatment plan can be chosen. Wounds need repair, and sometimes the wound needs to be opened so it can be cleaned. The treatment can be painful and it demands attention and effort—short-term success can lead to relapse if a treatment plan is not taken seriously.

"*The first goal* is simply to get you talking about the war experience we have identified together, so that we can identify what bothers you the most about it. Most warriors who go through the kinds of things you have experienced prefer not to talk about it, because thinking about it brings up painful feelings. So, they avoid thinking about it and talking about it. However, combat stress injuries are a little bit different than other sorts of injuries. For example, it's not like with a knee or an ankle injury where you come in, we do an X-ray of the area, and we figure out what's wrong and how to fix it. It would be nice if you could come in and we just do an X-ray of your brain and say, 'Oh, that's what's bothering you!' But we can't. The only way we know how to identify what is bothering you is to have you talk about it. When you are meeting with me, I'll ask you to talk in some detail about this war experience that is bothering you the most right now, which is an event that you feel like you can't get over or carry on from. Our job together will be to listen for what aspects of that experience might be making it most difficult for you to move on. We're going to talk about these experiences in a way that will help you adapt or adjust to the event and move forward more positively. I will be asking you questions to help you get clearer on not only what happened, but on what the event means to you, and how it has changed your thoughts and feelings about yourself, other people, and the world around you.

"After talking about the war event, *the second goal* is to help you to identify reactions that might be holding you back, and seeing whether there is any other way to think about and deal with the situation. Sometimes, when we experience something traumatic, we get very fixated on one aspect of the experience and start to interpret it in unhelpful and often inaccurate ways. While there may be some truth to the way you're interpreting things, often these beliefs become extreme and overgeneralized."

Here the therapist might use an example of helping a service member or veteran to modify unhelpful beliefs he or she had about his or her trauma experience. One example might be the following: "I was once working with a Marine who was a driver in motor transport. He was leading the convoy when his truck hit an IED. Since then, he has been saying to himself, 'I should have stopped the convoy', 'I should have slowed down', 'I should have scanned more'. A lot of 'shoulds' and self-blame. Through talking through the experience, he realized that he actually did everything that he could, and even did his job well that day. For example, he was a Lance Corporal so he wasn't going to be able to stop the convoy. He was not the only one in charge that day. He wasn't solely responsible for scanning the environment. No one else saw the IED either. However, he wouldn't have been able to see his experience in this other way if he hadn't talked it through."

> "Finally, *the third goal* is to help you to start reclaiming some of the good parts of yourself or good ways to see others and the world around you, and to accept but not be defined by some of the negative aspects of your deployment. For example, a lot of veterans say things like, 'I feel like I'm not the same person I used to be', or 'I can never be as relaxed, as fun, as close to others as I used to be'. Our job is to help you start to get back some of that person you used to be. Part of this may be learning to accept things that have happened, even if it is painful to do so. In other words, learning to live with the things that happened in the best way possible. For example, some service members and veterans feel upset about having killed people, feel that they didn't do their best in theater, or are upset about losing a buddy. Of course, I would love to just magically take away all of the pain from these experiences, but I can't. I can't change the fact that you killed someone or that your buddy's gone now. So it's looking at how these experiences are affecting you today, learning to accept them as best as possible, and figuring out how to live with them, as best as possible so that you have the future that you want to have. This therapy is designed to help veterans and service members pursue future possibilities that might seem 'off the table' right now."

WHAT GENERALLY TO EXPECT FROM ADAPTIVE DISCLOSURE

As we stated previously, it is critically important to provide the service member or veteran with accurate information about what to expect in the course of adaptive disclosure. In the case of loss or moral injury, this should include initial information about the experiential breakout components and what the patient will be asked to do during the imaginal dialogues. It is also important to give the patient a clear sense of what to expect as a result of therapy—that is, that it will not eliminate all the distressing things he or she has been experiencing.

> "Because we're just going to be meeting for a couple of months, it is important to realize that adaptive disclosure is not intended to fix all of the symptoms you are experiencing. Instead, we hope to provide you with an example of how coping with your experiences can look different when you talk about them, share them with somebody, and allow yourself to think about them and face them, rather than avoiding them. We hope that you'll come out of adaptive disclosure thinking and feeling differently about things, but we ask that you keep in mind that this is just the beginning of a longer process of sorting through and moving on from some of the difficult experiences you had in the military.
>
> "In addition to today's meeting, you and I will be meeting seven more times. The last meeting will be used to wrap-up, plan for the future, and get feedback about how this went. I would also like to get feedback from you about your experiences—what helped and what did not seem to hit the mark. I am going to ask you to fill out a very brief questionnaire at the beginning of each meeting to track how you are doing. Is that OK with you? Finally, I will be asking you to do some homework to try-on some of the things we will be discussing in between sessions. Do you have any thoughts or questions thus far?"

EDUCATING THE PATIENT ABOUT COMBAT AND OPERATIONAL STRESS INJURY, AND PTSD

The patient needs to hear about your working understanding of the causes of his or her suffering and the healing plan that should logically flow from this conceptualization. Any didactic information should be peppered with personalized information stemming from what the therapist has learned about the service member or veteran's principal military harm and the psychological, spiritual, social, and biological impact of that experience.

> "Although we will be tailoring the intervention to your personal experiences, it might be helpful to first discuss some general issues

about combat and operational stress injuries and PTSD. What have you been told about combat stress, and how does this fit with your own experience?"

Bear in mind that service members routinely get briefs or lectures about combat and operational stress injury. It is important to respect what the patient already knows and not to belabor the psychoeducational component. Use the following information to address any gaps in knowledge or inaccuracies:

"Would it be helpful to you to talk about combat stress injuries and where they come from (in a little more detail)?"

Here the therapist should use as discussion points the three principal harms or sources of combat stress to continue assessing the source of the patient's distress. The therapist can go through each one, discussing how they might fit for the patient. The exception to this would be discussion about doing things or failing to prevent things that violate a moral code of conduct. Here, the therapist should mention it as a source of combat stress with which many service members struggle and state that adaptive disclosure is a unique therapy, because it is in part designed to help people with these kinds of issues. However, at this point in therapy, the therapist should not push the patient to talk about his or her own possible experiences engaging in morally injurious behaviors, unless the service member provides the information on his own. Some patients may misperceive that a therapist is placing moral value judgments on combat actions or inactions if these issues are pursued too aggressively by the therapist. The therapist should refrain from encouraging such disclosures if the patient does not acknowledge them or is not yet ready to share them. We have found that some patients divulge such concerns later in therapy, once a level of trust and rapport with the therapist has been established. So simply noting at the outset of therapy that these issues can be dealt with in therapy is sufficient.

"Combat and operational stress injury can come from three sources:

1. *Life threat*: Being in dangerous situations in which your life was in danger or you were at risk of being severely injured can cause mental injury. Was there a time when you had a close call or thought that you would die? What was that like for you?

2. *Loss of life*: For most people, losing someone close to you is

one of the worst things that can happen. Did you lose any buddies over there?

3. *Moral injury*: Events that violate expectations about how someone should be treated or how things should go in war can be morally injurious. This is a common theme that we are seeing in our work with service members and veterans.

"For some, it is not the bullets flying or the IEDs, or even the loss of life. What haunts them are things they did or did not do, or things that others did, that violate deeply held beliefs about right and wrong. For example, people usually join the military because they strongly believe in what it stands for, and they internalize a code of conduct and system of values. But some service members find that things don't go according to a just and moral code of conduct, or they find themselves behaving in ways that make them feel shame and disgust. Other service members see others behave this way, or they see commanders make poor choices. For still others, seeing too much human suffering and death without being able to help or make a change can take a toll. Some talk about seeing all of the suffering in Iraq and Afghanistan: how women and children were treated and their way of living. They also talk about how difficult it is to see so much death and carnage and not be able to help. Any of these experiences can cause what we call 'moral injury.' This entails feeling demoralized, like losing your moral compass. This can cause you to feel shame and disillusionment, and to withdraw from others. Did anything like this happen for you?"

By explicitly mentioning violations of moral codes, therapists can impart the expectation that they are not threatened or averse to hearing about such experiences.

"Because deployment affects service members in all these various ways, no one exposed to combat is unaffected; no one comes out unchanged. Many of these changes can help you grow as a person, and in your military role (e.g., you become a better leader if you are tuned into what can be damaging to mental health in war). Yet other changes are damaging. Our job is to minimize the negative impact and maximize your opportunities for growth. What is important is to begin to navigate the changes that have occurred, to shape them in a more productive direction. First, we need to make a proper diagnosis of the key source of your injury and the nature of your difficulties."

SETTING UP THE FIRST EXPOSURE AND PROCESSING SESSION

The work required for an effective exposure therapy is significant. Therapists need to clarify for patients not only what will happen but also that it will not be easy, and it may be distressing, then to reassure patients that the process will be not only safe but also worthwhile.

> "Starting next week, I'll ask you to describe the event in detail—including your thoughts and reactions at the time—as well as how the event has affected you since then. Is that OK with you? Because this stuff is difficult to focus on, even though it might be upsetting, going back to it in your imagination, in the safety of our meeting, in this room, will allow you to get clear on the source of your injury and the meaning of the experience now, and what it might mean about how you see yourself moving forward in the future. Once we can assess that, we can talk about ways of helping you repair the wound and rehabilitate as you move forward as a service member, a family member, friend, and person. Does this make sense to you? What do you think that will be like for you?"

If the patient expresses considerable ambivalence and apprehension, it will be important to be confident and reassuring. The appropriate response is to normalize these reservations and note that most people find that working in this way winds up being less distressing than they had feared it would be. As described later in this book, there are ways to "titrate" exposure for maximal therapeutic effect—either by increasing emotional engagement for those who are too analytical or matter-of-fact, or decreasing emotional engagement of exposure for those having inordinate difficulty describing and discussing the traumatic event. Below, we provide heuristic narrative to introduce the work pertaining to loss and moral injury. A thorough treatment of exposure is provided in Chapter 7.

Loss Events

If the principal harm is a loss, also tell the patient the following:

"In addition to sharing your memory of this loss—when it happened or when you found out about it—I will be asking you to do something that at first may seem strange. I am going to ask you to have a conversation with the person you lost (use the person's name if you know it). I am going to ask you to share your current experiences in imagination with your eyes closed. If this goes well, though it may be painful for you, I think you will see that it is useful. I will walk you through this and help you throughout."

Morally Injurious Events

If the principal harm is a moral injury, also tell the patient the following:

"In addition to sharing your memory of this experience, I will be asking you to do something that at first may seem strange and difficult to imagine doing. I am going to ask you to have a conversation with someone in your past or present who cares for you deeply, someone who really always has your back. This person needs to be someone who is forgiving—who wants what is best for you and would not want you to suffer. I am going to ask you to share your experiences with this person with your eyes closed, using your imagination. I am going to ask you to have an actual conversation with this person. If this goes well, though it could be painful for you, I think you will see that it is useful. I will walk you through this and help you throughout. Between now and our next meeting, I want you to think about who this person should be. It could be a parent, a coach, a leader, a religious figure, a best friend."

THE MEANING AND IMPLICATION OF KEY EVENTS ASSIGNMENT

At the end of the first session, therapists should discuss the role of homework and assign The Meaning and Implication of Key Events Form (see Appendix 2). This form is similar to the *Impact Statement* used in cognitive processing therapy (Resick & Schicke, 1992) and is common to many trauma- or adversity-focused therapeutic approaches (e.g., Gortner, Rude, & Pennebaker, 2006). In adaptive disclosure, the goal is to establish a baseline of constructions and meanings that patients can use as a basis of comparison at the end of the therapy (they will be asked to fill out this form again before the last session). This is an assignment that they can choose to do on their own and report at the last meeting. It is an excellent way to start the dialogue about change or lack of change at the outset of the next session. Another goal is to get the patient in the right frame of mind for his or her first processing session (Session 2), to prime the psychological and emotional pump, if you will. It is not necessary that the patient share or read the written content, in part because questions about meaning and implication are asked at the end of the exposure phase of a given processing session. It is a nice gesture of empowerment to respect the patient enough to have him or her decide what to do with respect to sharing the content of this homework assignment, and keeping it private is perfectly legitimate. Nevertheless, if patients want to, or if the therapist thinks it will be helpful, the patient can read the narrative aloud at the start of Session 2 (or opt to have the therapist read the form). The aim is to empathize, reflect, and establish understanding.

> "Each week, I will usually have an assignment for you to complete. These assignments can help us get the most out of our work together. One thing is for sure, the real change in your life has to be outside these walls, so the homework is an attempt to kick-start that process.
>
> "This week, I am going to ask you to write about how you think about and explain the war (or military) experience we have agreed to work on in our next several meetings. If, after you leave today, you change your mind about the event that is currently most distressing for you, that is fine. Go with a different event instead. Just be sure you're choosing a different event because you've thought about it and the new event really is more bothersome to you. They key is not to change the event to something else just because it'll be easier to think and write about."

Some service members cringe when they hear the word "trauma" or "traumatic," or the terms become confused with physical trauma. For those service members, it is best not to use the term "trauma." In any case, ask the service member with whom you are working about his or her reaction to the terms you use. It will provide an important window into his or her world. Also, it is understandably difficult for some to choose a single traumatic event. In this situation, tell the patient that the selection of one event is not meant to diminish the impact or significance of any other memory. The goal is to find a way to start tackling a key important experience among many, to have a place to start your work together. The plan is that lessons learned about one experience generalize in positive ways to other war events.

Hand the patient "The Meaning and Implication of Key Events Form" (Appendix 2) and walk him or her through what the questionnaire is and what you need him or her to do for homework.

> "I want you to use what we call 'The Meaning and Implication of Key Events Form' to think and write about how this experience has changed you. I want you to think about how you have changed—how you are a different. The goals of adaptive disclosure are to clarify for you over time the meaning and implication of this experience in terms of your view of yourself, other people, and the world, then to examine and change the really damaging parts. Write as much as would be useful for you. It would be best if you could write one page about these important issues. I am going to ask you to do this task again at the end of our work together so you can compare where you are, then and now. The main goal for writing these things right now is to get you thinking about the meaning and implication of your military experience. I will be asking you questions about these matters the next time we meet; this form will help you feel prepared. Finally, if you think it would be helpful, you can read what you wrote the next time we meet.
>
> "You might find yourself wanting to avoid this assignment or to put it off as long as possible. However, in order for this assignment to be most helpful to you, try to start soon, so that you have enough time to say what you need to say. Pick a time and place where you have as much privacy as possible, so you can really pay attention to your thoughts and feelings while writing. Ideally, you should start today, while our meeting is still fresh in your mind. Do you have any questions?"

If the patients express concern about what they should say if someone they know sees them filling out the questionnaire, the therapist should role-play with the patients and model some options. This experience might also help the patients at other points in the therapy if they are particularly immersed and affected by adaptive disclosure and people inquire about what is going on.

Ideally, at this point, the patient has been assessed, is deemed appropriate for adaptive disclosure, understands what the therapy entails, and is ready for the first processing session described in Chapter

7. Also, at this point, the therapist knows the event that will start the processing and whether the event is a danger-based, a loss-based, or a moral injury.

SUMMARY

In this chapter, we have reviewed what clinicians need to do in the first adaptive disclosure session. This entails educating patients about what adaptive disclosure is, what will be required of them, and what the clinician will be doing. The goal is to provide accurate expectations about the therapy and to set the patient up, so that he or she hits the ground running in the next session.

CHAPTER 7

The Exposure Component

Active Treatment Sessions 2 to 7

Now that the patient understands the therapy and is on board, it is time to begin the focused processing of the principal harm. Each session begins with a raw imaginal, emotional processing of the trauma memory (exposure). This happens for any event type (danger/life threat, loss, or moral injury). The exposure component entails slowed, first-person, real-time immersive disclosure and uncovering of dreaded, charged, and salient aspects of the principal harm identified at the start of the treatment. Depending on the session and the event type, this lasts for 15–30 minutes. Unlike what takes place in prolonged exposure, for non-danger-based events, the disclosure is not repeated within the same session; rather, the goal is to engage in a single disclosure slowly enough to permit attention to detail and access to emotion. It is expected that fuller disclosure of the meaning and implication of the experience and associated emotion will progress over the course of the active treatment sessions.

In each session, the event processing is also followed by a period that allows the patient to return psychologically to the present and to share what the experience was like for him or her in an atmosphere of non-judgmental empathy and caring. This period is also designed to promote insight about the meaning and implication of the experience in the moment and foreseeing into the future. For fear-based life-threatening trauma, the exposure and postexposure dialogue is intended as a sufficient change agent. Because sound treatments already exist for danger-based, high fear traumas, we use a similar approach for these principal warzone harms. Adaptive disclosure diverges substantively for processing loss and moral injury. This chapter describes in detail the exposure component for all types of harms.

In the case of loss and moral injury, the exposure and postexposure dialogue is followed by the loss- and moral injury-related experiential techniques, respectively. These are described in detail in Chapter 8. The additional breakout strategies for loss and moral injury are designed to provide opportunities to help the patient unearth constructions of the meaning and implication of war zone harms, consider additional alternative and more helpful ways of thinking about his or her experience, and collaboratively identify a long-term path toward healing and recovery. In the case of grief or moral injury, the sessions should be broken down roughly in fourths (one-fourth of the therapy time each for exposure, postexposure dialogue, experiential strategies, and postexperiential dialogue). In the case of life-threatening trauma, after the check-in, the therapy session time can be broken roughly into halves. A flow chart of Sessions 2–7 is shown in Figure 7.1.

In some cases, clinicians will not have enough information to make a judgment about whether to follow the initial exposure and postexposure dialogue with a breakout experiential technique. In other words, they may not have enough information prior to the second session to make a judgment about whether the event constitutes a loss or a moral injury. Or clinicians may not be confident that the addition of an experiential technique is indicated, because the service member or veteran may not be sufficiently prepared. There may also be a general expectation that too much, too soon might not be a good idea. In these instances, clinicians should only do the exposure component plus the postexposure dialogue. Otherwise, if indicated, clinicians should use an experiential strategy for loss or moral injury, starting in Session 2.

DISCUSSING "THE MEANING AND IMPLICATION OF KEY EVENTS" ASSIGNMENT (SESSION 2)

After check-in (which entails determining how the patient is doing since the last meeting and asking whether he or she has any questions or needs clarification about the treatment), therapists should inquire about the writing task assigned at the end of the first session:

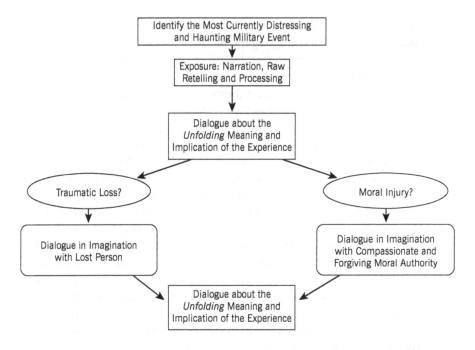

FIGURE 7.1. A flow diagram of adaptive disclosure, Sessions 2–7.

"When last we met, I asked you to identify an event that has been particularly difficult for you. I mentioned that we would be spending the next few sessions considering that experience in some detail—that we would examine not only the specifics of the event but also how it currently is affecting you currently and what kinds of things it causes you to think about. You indicated that you wanted to discuss (the specific event here). Is that the event you wrote about using the 'Meaning and Implication of Key Events Form'? What was this assignment like for you? What did you get out of it?"

As discussed at the end of Chapter 6, depending on the preferences of the patient and the exigencies of the case, the written account of the meaning and implication of the event can be read aloud or the patient can "hand it in" to be read aloud now by the therapist or be read by the therapist later. The goal is to honor the work completed and to establish an initial shared understanding of the event and its meaning and implication at the start of therapy. The therapist should also listen (or look for) clues about what is not said (avoided) and other conflict-laden and salient aspects that may need to be processed therapeutically. The therapist should be particularly attuned to changes in the patient's beliefs about the self, world, others, and his or her future as a result of the experience. The therapist should also listen for why the patient believes the event occurred, and what he or she believes was the cause of the event, with a focus on his or her unrealistic expectations or beliefs. If the patient did not complete the "Meaning and Implication of Key Events Form," the therapist should ask the patient to complete the assignment orally in session. The therapist should ask explicitly about the impact of the event on the patient's perceptions of self, others, the world, and the future. The therapist should use his or her own discretion to determine whether the form should be reassigned and reviewed the following week.

The event briefly described on the form needs to be seen as a starting place. The therapist should allow the patient to change the event to be used in therapy. Because the event generated in the last session was advanced "on the spot," he or she may have been able to identify a more fruitful event in the intervening week. The criterion is that the event should be the one that currently is most distressing and haunting, and an experience that has been difficult for the patient to come to terms with and confront.

EXPOSURE THERAPY COMPONENT: SESSION OVERVIEW

In adaptive disclosure, the exposure component is similar to well-published exposure therapy techniques and strategies. For additional resources, the reader is directed to the "prolonged exposure" therapy approach described by Foa and colleagues (Foa & Rothbaum; 2001; Foa et al., 2007; see *www.ptsd.va.gov/professional/continuing_ed/ prolonged_exposure.asp*). The assumption is that patients seeking treatment have insufficiently processed various war memories. Typically, intense aversive feelings and thoughts thwart focused and sustained processing, which prevents healing and recovery. In addition, avoidance maneuvers and defensive behaviors create collateral problems (e.g., pushing loved ones or peers away). The goal is to allow sustained engagement with something that would otherwise be avoided (e.g., a difficult combat memory), so that immobilizing appraisals can be identified, explored, and reconsidered. Because trauma survivors understandably attempt to avoid sustained consideration of the event and its implications, they are often unaware of tacit interpretations they have drawn, because the effect of the trauma has resulted in an impasse. Although such interpretations (e.g., "This will forever define me") are often based in reality and are accurate to a degree, they are frequently extreme and overgeneralized. Even worse, they may not be explicitly acknowledged or considered by the trauma survivor. It is only through sustained engagement (i.e., exposure) that the emotions surrounding trauma and related interpretations can be identified and reconsidered. In other words, patients need to "stay with the event" long enough for the beliefs to become articulated and explicitly discussed.

At the start, the therapist should describe what will happen:

> "I would like to help you process the experience you shared in our first session. Each week, I will ask you to close your eyes and imagine the event in detail. I am going to ask you to describe this thing that happened in the past as if it is happening now, again, while you imagine it. I want you to refer to yourself as 'I' and use the present tense as you share what happened. For example, instead of saying 'I opened the door,' I want you to say, 'I am open-ing the door.' I may ask you questions about the specifics of the event, including things you remember seeing, hearing, thinking, and doing. I'm going to try not to interfere or interrupt too much, though, because I want you to be able to relive the experience as fully as possible. By really connecting with the experience in ses-sion, it will be easier to understand how it has impacted you, and it will be easier to understand the meaning it has for you currently and how we might be able to understand it differently, so that you can move beyond it. So we'll start each session by discussing the details of the event and try to remember it in as much detail as possible. By doing so, we will be able to zero in more quickly on the aspects that are most difficult to deal with and identify more clearly what the event means for you.
>
> "It may be the case that thinking about _____ causes you to think about other upsetting experiences—even from other time periods in your life. That is perfectly natural. It will be impor-tant to try your best to stay with and focus on the event you've identified. It may be that processing the event we've discussed will help you understand and process those other experiences, too—or it may be that further work is required to address those experi-ences after the conclusion of our work together. But by focusing on a single event over the next few sessions, you will have an

opportunity to understand and begin to recover from that experience, which if all goes well can create a positive ripple effect in your life. To be clear, as we go through this process, if significant issues or concerns arise, or if you find it difficult to keep memories of other experiences at bay, please let me know. It may be that we need to discuss particularly pressing things further. But if you are not having great difficulty with those other experiences—if you just are reminded of them—we'll try to stick with the primary event that you've identified. Does that make sense? Do you have questions?"

Ideally, exposures are immersive—the patient is fully reliving the sights, smells, and felt experiences, as well as concurrent thoughts in real time. However, clinically, for some patients, it may be necessary to modify the impact of and engagement with the event. What is to be avoided is recounting that is matter-of-fact or done in an emotionally disengaged manner. Professionals who are unfamiliar with exposure therapy may fear patients' loss of control, intense affect, or dissociative reactions. Clinicians need to be confident that despite such understandable concerns, reliving can be therapeutic. Indeed, exposure therapy is underutilized in practice because of a lack of training and confidence in the approach (Becker, Zayfert, & Anderson, 2004). Professionals' concerns should be mollified by best-practice consensus guidelines for the treatment of PTSD that recommend exposure treatment (e.g., Foa et al., 2008). Confidence in exposure therapy is particularly important, because patients will be reluctant and readily perceive therapists' caution. Too much caution confirms patients' experience that sustained recall is dangerous and harmful, not only for them but for others. The goal of exposure therapy is to promote corrective experience, such as not having one's worst fears realized and instead experiencing relief, having someone provide caring support and understanding during a time of vulnerability, and meaning making. This cannot be accomplished unless the patient gives up (at least some) control, avoidance maneuvers, and inhibition, and he or she allows powerful feelings to surface. In adaptive disclosure, the added assumption is that because of the unprecedented and raw nature of the experience, exposure can uncover or reveal previously vague or unappreciated elements of the trauma memory, and new feelings and associations.

When the principal harm is a highly fearful, life-threatening experience, the immersive aspect of the exposure component is particularly important. The goal is to process fully all aspects of the memory and to experience sustained high levels of fear, in order to promote extinction of conditioned fear and expose patients to the new learning that arises when they experience within- and between-session decrements in fear. Furthermore, through sustained exposure, patients who have experienced the threat of annihilation or other grave dangers develop awareness that emotions surrounding the trauma memory—though intensely aversive—are tolerable and do not persist indefinitely. The intent and goals of the exposure component are very different if the principal harm is loss or moral injury.

In the context of loss and moral injury, the exposure component is necessary but not sufficient. Sadness and guilt from loss, shame and self-loathing from personal transgression, or anger about others' moral transgression, cannot be extinguished by repeated intensive processing. For these principal harms, the goal of the exposure is to help patients to disclose the events in detail, experience raw feelings, and reveal their emerging narrative about the meaning and implication of the events. This information is used to start the experiential components for both loss and moral injury.

Assessing Intensity of Aversive Emotions during Exposures

When patients are processing a memory during the exposure component, therapists should find a way of monitoring patients' overall distress in a nonintrusive manner. In many instances, a simple question such as "How are you doing?" might suffice. In other contexts, it may help to teach the patient the Subjective Units of Distress Scale (SUDS), which is standard practice in exposure therapy. Originally, the SUDS was used in the context of fear-based problems and phobias, to ensure that a high degree of arousal and negative affect was present in-session, which is a prerequisite to extinction over the course of a given session and across sessions. Because in-session extinction is not necessarily the goal of treatment in modern variants of exposure therapy for PTSD, SUDS ratings have become more of a clinical guide to emotional engagement. This quick-gist assessment of distress and the intensity of negative affect may help to provide feedback that the therapist can use to modify the process. If the SUDS ratings are low, then the patient is not focusing on the right details, or he or she is using defensive maneuvers that thwart the triggering of painful emotions and states of vulnerability. If therapists choose to use SUDS ratings, the SUDS should be introduced as follows:

"Periodically, while your eyes are closed, I'd like you to give me a number from 0–100 to describe how upset you are, where 0 = *not at all upset* and 100 = *as upset as you can imagine.* This will help us track what is going on for you, without getting too much in the way."

Postexposure Dialogue

"Most experienced exposure therapists acknowledge that the post-exposure conversation is often the most impactful and therapeutic element of exposure therapy. This is not surprising. By design, the exposure puts patients into a poignant state of mind, and the expression of intense feelings and raw thoughts creates a charged, intimate atmosphere and bond between patient and therapist. The therapist not only bears witness to the disclosed horrific experiences with intensive focal empathy (the observer in participant–observer), but he or she also engages in and directs the process (the participant) in a way that dials him or her into where the patient is and makes him or her sensitive to the patient's needs when emerging from the exposure and upon opening his or her eyes. If all goes well, the patient will be in a state that motivates him or her to share and to receive feedback—this is a hot cognitive state of mind that can be leveraged therapeutically. It is powerful and healing to feel understood and nurtured by someone who witnesses your suffering in a non-judgmental manner."

We provide a series of specific instructions to guide the postexposure dialogue at the end of this chapter. To some extent, therapists need to *go with their guts* about where to start the postdisclosure dialogue. The initial goals are to help patients recover a sense of being in the now, shore up their vulnerability; nurture a reflective and sharing frame of mind, and communicate empathy and understanding of what took place during the exposure. Sometimes it is helpful to take the reins at the start, while the patient is recouping. This can be accomplished by sharing what the experience was like using reflective statements and personal observations (e.g., "That was intense; you did such a good job staying with it. It seemed like there was a point when it really hit you hard. How are you doing right now and what was this like for you?").

Eventually, the following topics should be covered in the dialogue:

- Ask the patient whether it went the way he or she thought it would, and whether bad things happened (according to his or her expectations). In most cases, when asked, the patient acknowledges that although the exposure was difficult, it was more manageable than anticipated. In the comparatively rare instances when patients report that the exercise was as difficult as they had expected, therapists can still provide positive feedback to patients for being able to do something so difficult, emphasizing that it does get more manageable with time and that the first couple of exposures are always the most difficult. Stated differently, therapists can make it clear that patients have already faced and tolerated the most difficult phase and can promote the expectation that each time will become slightly more manageable than the time before.

- Determine what the patient learned from the experience.

- Determine which parts of the memory were most difficult to stay with and which parts the patient may have avoided or "fast forwarded" through. Eventually emphasize that the parts of the memory that the patient most wants to avoid are usually the most important parts of the memory to stay with, and agree to try to connect with those aspects of the memory for a longer duration during the next exposure. The therapist should take note of which aspects of the memory were most difficult for the patient, and should help the patient stay with that aspect of the memory during the next exposure, for example, by asking numerous questions relating to that aspect of the memory during the exposure to make sure that they do not move through it too quickly.

- Discuss the meaning and implication of the experience just processed. This needs to be seen as an emerging and dynamic narrative. This should initially be queried without use of specific prompts. If the patient has difficulty identifying meaning and implication, the therapist may then ask whether the event causes the patient to think differently about him- or herself relative to his or her sense of self prior to deployment. The patient may also be asked about perceptions of others, the world, and the future.

This aspect of the postexposure dialogue is particularly critical and necessary. In the context of a life-threatening harm, the goal is to use Socratic questioning to provide opportunities to counter catastrophic expectancies about safety and beliefs about incompetence and personal failure. In the context of loss and moral injury, the goal of the exposure component is to unearth meaning dimensions and to acknowledge them. For these principal harms, it is no less important to discuss the meaning and implication of the events after the exposure. However, for loss and moral injury, critical Socratic questioning is not used to promote therapeutic meaning making at this stage. This is done after the therapeutic dialogue with the person who died (for loss) or a compassionate forgiving moral authority (for moral injury). The reader will recall that in adaptive disclosure, the goal is to use patients' constructions of what these figures think about their damning conclusions and to voice what they want for themselves moving forward in their lives. Nevertheless, as the reader will see in Chapter 8, the therapist also uses a Socratic dialogue after the therapeutic dialogue to maximize the potential for accommodating this new healing and forgiving information.

Ending the Session

Therapists should ask patients what they think they will take with them from the session. Additionally, the therapist should discuss the potential possibility of symptoms and painful thoughts and feelings being stirred up by the session, noting that this should abate over time. Patients should be reminded that any potential increases in symptoms are not a sign that the treatment "isn't working" but rather that important and necessary work ("cleaning the wound") is being done. The therapist can say:

> "What do you think you will take from today's session to think about throughout the week? What really stood out for you? I know this was difficult and more than likely you will continue to think about it from time to time throughout the week. This is very normal. Sometimes we find that as patients start to look at difficult experiences they've had, they initially experience more unwanted thoughts about the experience than they had been experiencing previously. This will go away with time."

The therapist should also assess the patient at the end of the session to make sure his or her acute distress has dissipated. If not, he or she should inquire about what helps reduce these experiences. The therapist encouraged these natural coping behaviors or introduces grounding or relaxation techniques prior to ending the session (see Appendix 3, "Calming and Attention-Focusing Techniques").

EXPOSURE COMPONENT: SPECIFIC INSTRUCTIONS

As stated, therapists should foster as much emotional experiencing and sharing as possible. They need to use their personal, relational, and technical skills to foster a safe, comfortable, charged atmosphere, and they must be active and engaged. If the quality of the relationship is sound and the patient is responsive and capable, the therapist should push, prompt, cue, direct, redirect, and even prod. Therapists should respectfully try to test the limits of the patient's ability to process events and focus on the emotions they trigger. In many instances, during exposure, therapists need "not to take no for an answer," because if given the option, most patients would not want to be vulnerable or share deeper meanings and darker aspects of experience.

However, an assumption about exposure therapy is that at least some sustained, frank, and focused sharing of troubling war zone memories is better than none and can be therapeutic. This is chiefly because even brief and superficial conscious processing is otherwise avoided (and typically not shared) and if negative and catastrophic expectations are disconfirmed in a session and over several sessions, the motivation to avoid (or dismiss) recalling trauma memories will be reduced. In theory, revisions in expectations (new learning) lead to better monitoring, planning, preparation, and reduced reactivity to situations that trigger recall of painful war-related memories. So, if a patient resists expressing certain feelings or experiencing a depth or intensity of feeling, accept that limitation without giving up on the general goal of engaging with and processing trauma. Instead, focus on content, meaning, and what the patient sees as the implication of the experience in terms of how he or she feels about him- or herself, others, and what he or she expects from him- or herself and people generally while moving forward in his or her life. Bear in mind that if a patient seems not to want to cross a line of sharing disclosure with the therapist, perhaps because of the briefness of their work together, it does not necessarily mean that he or she does not have moments of deep feeling or that there will never be occasions when he or she reaches a depth of feeling when recalling various combat traumas.

Therapists need to be keenly engaged participant–observers. They need to listen and watch for changes in behavior (movement, shallow rapid breathing, tears, etc.), and affect, especially facial expressions. These are the cues that the memory processing is on the right track. On the one hand, exposure therapy requires therapists to be patient and respectful of the patient in the driver seat, sharing what he or she deems to be sufficient details of the experience. In this primary role, the therapist's job is patiently to shape and encourage the patient to focus and sustain his or her attention on the real-time reliving experience *as controlled and narrated by the patient.*

On the other hand, therapists at times are also required to be quite directive. For example, it is often necessary to tell patients to get back to aspects of a traumatic experience to which they have alluded but not focused on. Sometimes therapists also need to direct patients to go "beyond the information given" and explore previously avoided aspects of traumatic experiences and their implications. The art is found in hypothesizing what is being left out from a trauma narrative. This requires the therapist to remain open to and aware of the elements of the memory that may be avoided, or to parts of the narrative that seem incongruent or not sufficiently fleshed out. When done well, this process is flowing and dynamic, taking into account the personality of the patient and the quality of the therapeutic relationship. The therapist must be intuitive but not overly presumptuous, testing the patient's emotional response to different aspects of the memory, and learning what must be approached more fully, all the while being empathically present and seeking collaboration in decision making with the patient. At times, this process may seem counter to the natural desire to ease the patient's suffering, so the clinician must be vigilant for urges to back away and the subtle ways these urges this may be manifest. Of course, the exposure work is immeasurably difficult for the patient, and requires courage and trust that the pain is worth the gain. To a much smaller but important degree, this is also true for the therapist.

Directing patients to conflict-laden elements that may be avoided or unacknowledged should be done judiciously. It is important that therapists to be balanced and not too heavy handed, that they not direct attention to themselves or inadvertently behave in a manner perceived as disrespectful. Yet it is worth pointing out, especially to therapists who are not directive in their work, that if direction and suggestion is done in the context of a good therapeutic relationship, the worst that can happen is that the patient does not respond or gets a little annoyed. This can be fertile ground for discussion after the exposure session, so that the therapist can explain his or her intention and bolster the patient's agency by being respectful and collaborative.

To encourage hypothesis generation and assist in planning future exposure sessions and experiential breakouts, therapists should have a notepad with them during the exposure component to take notes about content and process. They should also jot down any nascent hypotheses about the themes and meanings that may need special attention during exposure.

Starting the Exposure Process

Well prior to beginning an exposure session, therapists need to be confident that the service member or veteran understands what is going to happen and why it is useful. They should then begin by saying:

> "If you're willing, I'd like you to close your eyes and recall and imagine (*be specific about the event*) as vividly as you can. I want you to tell me what is happening every step of the way. I want to hear what was happening before, during, and after (*the specific event*). I want you to tell me about it in the present tense, as if it were happening right now. This is important, but it will be awkward at first. I want you to use the words 'I am' and 'he or she is' to put you there, but in the here and now."

Many patients have difficulty adhering to use of the first-person present tense during their account. It is not crucial that they do so in order to obtain benefits from the exposure; if they keep talking in past tense after one or two gentle attempts to correct them, do not force the issue.

> "Try to include details on two different levels: what's going on outside of you, in terms of what you can see, hear, smell, taste, and feel, then what's going inside of you, in terms of what you feel inside your body (e.g., *your heart racing, or feeling cold or nauseated*) and also how you're feeling emotionally (*tense, sad, scared, horrified, angry, etc.*). Focusing on how you are feeling is especially important. Finally, I want you to slow this down; it is critical not to rush through this."

Patients may skip over or "fast-forward" through the worst aspects of the memory.

The following are basic questions to ask while conducting exposure therapy to direct patients' attention to different elements of a trauma memory in the first-person present tense, which is the prescribed mode to maximize engagement:

> "What are you seeing (sensing, smelling, or hearing)?"
>
> "What are you feeling (now) as you are seeing (hearing, smelling, etc.) _____?"
>
> "What comes to mind as you feel _____?"

Therapists should be artful about these prompts and include various nuances and specific elements that the patient is sharing into their queries. The more personalized and natural the prompts, the better the exposure. Prompt questions that can be useful include the following:

"Where are you, what is going on around you?"

"What do you see?"

"What are you hearing?"

"What can you smell?"

"What is going through your mind as you see these things?"

"What are you feeling emotionally? How does it feel?"

"What are you doing?"

"What is your job (or role) in this situation?"

"What is expected of you in this situation?"

Therapists should provide support and encouragement throughout the narrative. The following are some things that therapist might say to encourage the patient during the exposure therapy:

"I know this is difficult, you're doing a great job. Stay with this, I know how hard this is for you . . . "

As stated earlier, the therapist should be as directive as he or she needs to be—asking as many questions as necessary to get the patient to slow down and share details of the experience and his or her reactions to it. Issues to bear in mind include the following:

• Direct the exposure processing in a serial time frame. In other words, start with what was going on prior to the event, then the event itself, and on to later experiences, after the hell and panic of the moment was gone. This latter feature is very important. For example, if there was a severe injury or death in a firefight or an explosion, the patient is caught up in the moment of doing his or her job and securing safety or returning fire that he or she does not have time to reflect and process. Once he or she gets back to a secure area, hours later (or perhaps even months later), he or she may reflect. These moments are very important.

• Be sure to elicit details of not only the triggering event but also the patient's specific reactions to the event at the time, including physical, emotional, cognitive, and behavioral responses.

• Therapists need to watch for excessive *military mission-speak*, which is service members or veterans speaking as if the conversation is about mission strategies and tactics. Redirect the patient to what happened and his or her responses to it, and probe for emotions and real-time constructions.

• Ask the patient to tell you who the characters are; names are highly evocative cues. For example, a therapist may ask the patient to tell him or her the names of the men/women in his or her squad. To promote vivid recall, therapists should ask patients whether they can see so-and-so's face right now, what he or she looks like, what he or she is like, and what he or she is doing?

Therapists need to develop an understanding of the key, high-probability psychological, spiritual, social, and biological sequelae of each principal military harm (danger-based events, losses, and moral injuries), and the emotions experienced as a result of reactivating memories of them during the exposure. The following is a general guide and starting place:

• If the predominant emotion is fear (and anticipatory anxiety), assume that the experience entails unpredictability, helplessness, vulnerability, a lack of control, and perhaps a lack of preparation and planning. It would also be worthwhile to hypothesize that the service member or veteran suffers from shame about underfunctioning during and after the life-threatening event and as a result of various PTSD symptoms since.

• If the predominant emotion is sadness, assume that the loss event also entails thoughts about personal failure to save the other, failure of events to conform to expectations about war, guilt about surviving, and a need to suffer. In all likelihood, the patient may have toxic metacognitions about this emotional reaction. Patients may deem themselves to be less strong and capable in their professional roles or less "manly" by virtue of tearfulness and sadness accompanying their memories.

• If the predominant emotion is anger as a result of the moral transgression of others (see Chapter 8), therapists should assume that the event was a violation of expectations of fairness, justice, and right and wrong, and poor leadership and command decisions. In these contexts, patients will understandably focus on what others have done. Consequently, it is difficult for them to focus on the *personal* meanings and implications of the experience. The challenge is to shift eventually to these matters, which are the only ones that are within the patient's control.

• If the predominant emotion is shame as a result of personal moral transgression (commission or omission; see Chapter 8), therapists should assume that the patient has absorbed all of the responsibility and culpability for a given act, feels evil and wonders whether he or she will taint others close to them, and feels unforgiven and unforgiveable. These experiences can result in a fundamental alteration in identity—from a just and good agent to a person forever defined by a reprehensible act. Needless to say, the journey back to a sense of worth and a life of purpose can be slow and arduous. Gradually separating a single act—no matter how salient—from the totality of self and promoting the consideration of reengaging with premorbid values and actions will be demanding but critically important tasks in adaptive disclosure and over the lifespan for many.

Because service members tend to highly value self-control in all spheres, the therapist should look especially for evidence of loss of control of behavior, emotions, or thinking during or after an event. Do not jump to conclusions about the significance of a loss of control, but if it seems connected with painful emotions, help the patient verbalize his or her specific response to the challenges of the event meant to him or her, both at the moment and subsequently. The patient may not even have noticed losing control, or he or she may have considered it par for the course. On the other hand, the patient may be left with a deep sense of failure, remorse, or shame because of what he or she did or failed to do at a crucial moment.

POTENTIAL PROBLEMS WITH EXPOSURE COMPONENT
Insufficient Emotional Engagement

Many patients recount the narrative in a matter-of-fact way in the wake of the traumatic experience, and may lapse into "giving a statement" (i.e., emotional avoidance). This can be limited by using the first-person present tense during the exposure component. If the patient has been reluctant to do so, encouraging himor her to close his or her eyes and visualize the scene may also be helpful. The therapist should remind the patient to use the present tense when describing the event and be more active in probing for sensory details and peritraumatic thoughts and feelings. Make sure that the patient fully understands why it is important to connect with his or her emotions during the exercise. If underengagement remains a problem, it may also be useful to revisit any fears the patient might have about feeling or showing emotion in session, which may be making him or her purposely shy away from emotional content.

Excessive/Overwhelming Emotional Engagement

It may be that the patient is surprised by the intensity of emotion that accompanies the recounting of an event that was deemed to be "manageable." If the level of processing seems too immersive and too intense, the therapist should remain calm, be supportive, and convey confidence that he or she will be able to handle, and help the patient to handle, whatever comes up. The therapist provides encouraging comments throughout and encourages the patient to continue with the narrative. He or she may suggest that the patient keep his or her eyes open and recount the event in past tense, which may render it more tolerable. The therapist may choose not to probe as much for sensory details. He or she should keep in mind that the goal of the exposure component is to get the patient emotionally aroused enough to allow for some hot cognitive processing. If the patient is doing this without recalling all aspects of the trauma, then this is sufficient. For patients who are highly engaged to the point that the exposure component feels counterproductive, the therapist can do a modified exposure, in which he or she engages in what looks more like a conversation about the trauma with the patient. For example, the therapist would still go through the exposure but in a conversational manner, by asking questions and responding to comments made by the patient.

In the highly unlikely event that the patient loses control and becomes so distressed by his or her recounting of the event that he or she demonstrates physical, cognitive, or emotional loss of control (e.g., perspiring profusely, shaking visibly, experiencing dissociation, becoming physically agitated, or raising his or her voice in rage), use behavioral calming techniques such as deep, slow diaphragmatic breathing to reduce physiological and mental arousal, then gently and carefully process with the patient the meaning of the symptoms during the session. None of these symptoms would be considered "normal" by the average patient. In discussing what happened, use the following strategies:

• Draw the patient's attention to what happened and ask if something similar has happened in the past, either during or after the event he or she has discussed. This might reveal a connection to an earlier childhood trauma.

- Be supportive and directive. Educate the patient that loss of normal control of one's body, thoughts, or emotions is a common symptom of a combat stress injury, just as loss of normal function of an arm or a leg is a normal symptom of a physical injury to that part of the body.

- Reassure the patient that loss of control was no more his or her fault than would be a limp if he or she had a sprained ankle or broken leg, or difficulty firing his or her weapon if he or she had an injured hand. But just like such physical injuries, stress injuries can heal. Therapy sessions can be thought of as being similar to physical therapy for an injured leg or arm: They can be painful and draw attention to the wounded body part, but they also help to promote healing.

Excessive Anger

A patient may become very angry and begin to ruminate on aspects of the narrative. It should be noted that for life-threatening trauma, the exposure component may not be as effective when the primary response is anger or rumination. In this context, hypothesize that the patient is avoiding feeling vulnerable and encourage him or her to focus on the parts of the narrative that elicit other affects. For other principal harms, therapists need to be mindful that anger is often an appropriate response when the patient felt (feels) violated in some way. Allow the anger to manifest, but also move to affects that underlie the anger: vulnerability, betrayal, sadness, and so forth, if possible. An example of a possible therapeutic approach to processing such difficulties is as follows:

> "We need to talk some about how you are responding to what is coming up around _____. First, what are your thoughts about what is coming up each time we talk about _____, have you noticed anything? It is becoming clear to me that once you start to get really pissed, it dominates things and pushes out other feelings you might be having. I certainly understand why you get angry—the thing that happened is such a raw deal, things did not go the way they should have, this kind of thing is not supposed to happen, it is like a betrayal. Do you know what I mean? Anger is a normal emotion and it often provides us with useful information—about things that we need to take action on.

Sometimes it can be excessive, though, and prevent us from being able to process an event and move forward. It's also sometimes easier to feel anger than to deal with other bad feelings you might be having, such as feeling sad, or scared, or guilty. If you stick with your anger and let it dominate you, you will have a hard time recovering, because, in order to heal, you need to feel all the feelings. I wonder if you would be willing to dig deeper and move beyond the anger. Can I get your permission to stop you when it seems to dominate you, so we can explore other things that might be going on?"

Service members and veterans tend to be comfortable with aggression (they are selected and trained to be), and they may tend to convert other affects into aggression as a way to manage them. However, unless they are sociopathic (a very small minority) they also tend to be comfortable with feelings of warmth and affection, especially toward peers. Most patients will quickly see how anger that is out of control is damaging the important relationships in their lives, as well as their careers.

PROCESSING APPRAISALS AND MEANINGS FOLLOWING EXPOSURE

As detailed earlier, the first 15–30 minutes of the session (the formal exposure component) is designed to make the distressing principal harm as salient as possible, in order to activate appraisals and interpretations of the event (including expectations for the future as a result of the event), such that these may be readily identified and processed throughout the remaining part of the session. For loss and moral injury, the goal in processing beliefs is not to disabuse the patient of problematic or distress-maintaining beliefs (at this stage). These beliefs may be fairly entrenched and may often be at least partially rational. The following are the goals of the postexposure dialogue:

- Make the beliefs explicit and articulated.
- Shed light on the degree to which the beliefs might be extreme and the patient may not be considering other possible explanations.
- Encourage the consideration of less absolute/rigid/self-damning appraisals.

The aim is to "plant healing seeds." The approach is not designed to supplant "irrational" thought with "rational" thought as in formal cognitive therapy (although this may occur). Instead, the goal is to encourage the mere consideration of other possible interpretations, some of which may be less "rational" but are nevertheless more adaptive. Furthermore, as an endpoint of this intervention, it is not necessary for the patient to arrive at the most logical and rational interpretation of his or her experience. Rather, the endpoint is to chip away at fixed and absolutist or rigid interpretations that create severe impairment and misery.

Another important goal of postexposure processing is to assess the meaning of the event and (if not known already) to determine whether a breakout experiential exercise focused on moral injury/betrayal or grief should become a focus of treatment (if not known a priori). Immediately following the exposure component, the therapist's task is to inquire about the meaning of the event. This dialogue should touch on themes that were identified on the Meaning and Implication of Key Events Form (at least as a starting place). The therapist should ask additional broad questions designed to elicit the patient's understanding of the event, why it is so difficult for him or her, and what it might mean for him or her moving forward in life. Questions should be purposely open/broad at the outset of this dialogue so that meaning and interpretations are not imposed by the therapist. In all likelihood, however, the questions need to become more focused and directive as the dialogue proceeds, especially if the patient is having difficulty identifying why this event is so troubling in terms of future and current adjustment. More focused questions will be informed by knowledge of themes and appraisals that are common to war-related distress, as well as by observations made by the patient during or immediately following the exposure component. In all likelihood, it will not be necessary to inquire about all of these domains in succession. The therapist should have some informed inclinations based on the assessment, as well as themes that emerged during the exposure component. Accordingly, the examples below of possible queries or themes are for illustrative purposes. It is *not* expected that all will be asked in order, like a structured clinical interview.

> "That sounds like a pretty terrible experience—and it's understandable why it continues to be so haunting. I'm wondering if you have thoughts about what this event means for you— both in terms of your reaction to it and relative to what it might mean for you as you move forward in your life?"

"What about this event is particularly difficult—relative to other tough combat and operational situations?"

"What was the worst thing about it?"

More detailed examples will be informed by the nature of the event described by the patient. For instance, if relevant:

"Were you particularly close with this person?"

"Was this the closest you came to losing your own life?"

"Did you feel that you didn't live up to your own expectations in that situation?"

"What does it mean to you—right now—that you find this experience so difficult?"

"What were some of your expectations about war prior to deploying? What did you think it would be like, and how did you think you would handle it?"

"Many service members (or veterans) I've talked to say that they are really excited about deploying. They have this idea that it is going to kind of be like a game, and this idea that while, of course, they *could* die, they won't. They say it's not usually until that first time in theater when they get shot at or lose a buddy that they realize the seriousness of war. And suddenly it's less fun. Many even say that they wanted to go home in that moment. Did that kind of thing happen to you at all?"

"Did this experience cause you to think differently about yourself or have a different opinion about who you are as a person compared to how you were before deployment? If so, how?"

These questions are designed to begin to make salient the "meta-meaning" of the event for the patient. The patient may have been so focused on details and emotions surrounding the event that he or she is unaware of unrealistic precombat expectations surrounding the ability to emerge from combat emotionally unscathed. One potential source of distress is feeling like a failure as a patient based on expectations that one should be able to handle any combat experience and move on. Lingering, intense distress may be rooted in this unrealistic precombat expectation. Does the patient believe that his or her emotional difficulty is incompatible with being a good patient? Is it possible to have performed to expectations (assuming this is true) and also be distressed? To get at these appraisals, the therapist might ask: What are your concerns about how this experience might impact you in the future? Do you believe it will continue to impact your functioning as a (Sailor, Airman, Soldier, or Marine—or as a husband, father, etc.)?

The issue here is whether the patient is conceptualizing the distress as a difficult but transient phenomenon—or whether the patient believes that he or she is forever marked or impaired by this experience. Therapeutic response and processing seek to strike a balance between unrealistic expectations to put the event behind forever and never be affected by it on the one hand, and being forever impaired and damaged by it on the other. Asking questions designed to foster an appreciation of the extreme and dichotomous nature of these positions, and designed to introduce consideration of a more reasonable middle ground will likely be fruitful. Ultimately, the patient needs to recognize that this event will always be a part of his or her history that is difficult/upsetting to think about, but that it need not fully define or incapacitate him or her. *We want patients to leave adaptive disclosure with the belief that it is possible to begin to move forward—shaped by the event but not dominated or completely defined by it.* Questions that get at these issues include "Do you feel like a fundamentally different person compared to how you were before the war as a result of this experience, and if so, how so?"

At this point, if the patient is having trouble articulating differences, or if he or she feels a bit stymied, the therapist can mention possibilities based on discrepancies noted from the pretreatment assessment. Again, it may be that the patient has beliefs that are grounded in reality—that are true to a degree but overgeneralized or extreme. Only through explicit discussion might it become apparent how extreme some of the patient's implicit beliefs are. This process may also be fruitful in causing the patient to consider other possibilities. A question that can be asked to prompt reflection about these matters is "Do you believe, or are you worried that, some life outcomes and goals may no longer be possible for you as a result of this experience?"

If we could, we would want service members and veterans harmed by war traumas to reclaim the person they were at the peak of their military service, as well as how potent, hopeful, and positive they may have been. Therapists need to appreciate that this is rarely possible. The goal should be to accommodate new experiences without being fully defined by them and be hopeful that the future can be better. When discussing the meaning and implication of the event processed in terms of expectations of the future, it is useful to get the patient to suspend judgment about what are typically firm dark conclusions. It is not necessary (or even possible) to fully disabuse the patient anyway. The desired process is to hold the patient's conclusions as one conceivable outcome while considering that the intervention and the passage of time might allow for outcomes that do not seem possible at present. If the "impossibility" of future desired outcomes is a foregone conclusion in the mind of the patient, it becomes a self-fulfilling prophecy. The goal of adaptive disclosure is not to eradicate painful memories and associations; this is not possible in any form of psychotherapy. Rather, we want the patient to question the conviction with which their dark conclusions are held, to consider that his or her feelings may change and that those feelings (though understandable) may not relate to what he or she can accomplish in the future.

To start processing shame and guilt, the therapist should ask: "Are there things about your experience that you find you cannot forgive yourself for? Either things that you did or things that you didn't do but wish you had?" If extreme guilt/shame is present, refer to the relevant breakout component in Chapter 8. Self-forgiveness will be difficult to achieve in the context of a brief intervention, but this section provides guidance for beginning that work. Even if guilt/shame is not extreme, the therapeutic dialogue will need to focus on the clarity of hindsight and the lack of such clarity before the outcome is known (assuming that this is true). Furthermore, making salient the barriers to acting in the desired manner at the time—especially given that the outcome was not known—can be helpful. Finally, identification of all persons and contributing factors—and formal allocation of degree of responsibility to each of these persons/factors—is a useful technique in helping the patient appreciate that he or she alone was not 100% responsible (again, assuming this is true—there may be exceptions). While it may not fully eradicate self-blame, this exercise can temper the degree of self-blame and can result in increased awareness of other contributing factor(s). Importantly, this exercise is packaged with discussion of forgiveness and activities related to making amends (see Chapter 8). Reassigning blame alone is insufficient and possibly inappropriate for guilt and shame from acts of commission or omission that entail culpability from the service member's point of view given military training and the requirements of battle. Consequently, adaptive disclosure gives the military culture a place in the therapy room, places validity in the voice of the service member, accepts a range of culture-consistent culpability, and targets damage to moral identity by focusing on moral repair (see Chapter 8).

Finally, in discussions of the meaning and implication of principal harms, therapists should look for opportunities to educate their patients about stress that is severe enough in either intensity or duration to inflict injuries to the mind or brain of anyone. The symptoms of a stress injury, just like the symptoms of a physical injury, are not in the individual's personal control, and are therefore never the individual's personal fault. Stress injury symptoms may include temporarily (or recurrently, after the event is over) losing the ability to stay calm and in control, or to perform in every way as desired and expected. The patient cannot be blamed for these symptoms, but as with physical injury symptoms, patients are responsible for attending to these symptoms, taking care of them, and getting further help if they do not resolve over time. Having stress injury symptoms never means a person is weak, but acknowledging them is always a sign of strength, and a reason for hope for the future.

HOMEWORK ASSIGNMENTS

Homework is really useful because it provides opportunities to extend the therapy work and start the necessary process of doing things differently *in vivo* over time. There may be legitimate push-back from patients about homework assignments because of their age, lifestyle, and culture, and their work and training (for service members) demands. Consequently, therapists need to use good judgment about whether homework assignments are feasible. In every case, it is important to probe and to attempt to test the limits of expressions of incredulity (or outright refusal) about homework. Referring to homework as "outside practice" might help. It is important to be clear about the value of working on various issues and trying out new ways of relating or behaving in the 99% of the time that occurs in-between sessions. However, failure experience, disappointment, and counterreactions of disengagement and distrust need to be avoided at all costs. Homework needs to be discussed at length, and ideas need to be generated collaboratively and collegially. Homework should always have clear goals related to the work being done in adaptive disclosure and be agreed upon; potential obstacles to its completion should be discussed (and problem-solved in advance). In other words, the homework should be meaningful, doable, and owned by the patient. Homework assignments can be written, behavioral, or simply issues to think about for the next meeting. The therapist needs to make sure to go over the assignment in the next session. In each instance, homework needs to be respected and honored (and reinforced). In terms of generating ideas for homework, the therapist might ask any of the following questions:

- "What do you think would be useful for you to do before our next session?"

- "What would you be willing to try to work on during the week?"

- "What kind of practice assignment seems doable for you to work on in the next week?"

Examples of homework assignments in the treatment of loss and moral injury are provided in Chapter 8. Here, we provide examples of homework options for life-threatening trauma and experiences of fear, hypervigilance, and vulnerability. For example, patients can write (or agree to think) about the following:

"What do you think might happen if you allow yourself to be vulnerable/emotional/trusting with others?"

"What do you think might happen if you allowed yourself to fully remember the event?"

"Who do you feel comfortable letting your guard down with? How much emotion can you show him or her? What types of things do you feel more comfortable sharing with him or her? What things do you keep to yourself even with this person and why?"

"What are the costs and benefits of being on guard too much? How might too much vigilance negatively affect you at work and at home?"

"How likely is it that the negative events that you're guarding against and watching for might actually happen? How often have they happened to you before?"

"What is the difference between being vigilant and excessively vigilant?"

Therapists should also assign homework that entails *in vivo* exposure to avoided trigger contexts, because they trigger fear and recall of life-threatening experiences. A patient might be asked to do the following:

- Create a hierarchy of events from least challenging to most challenging, and have the patient start with the least challenging exercise and work his or her way up the hierarchy (e.g., going to the store at increasingly busy periods, working his or her way toward sitting increasingly toward the middle of the movie theater, or gradually decreasing the number of times he or she is allowed to check for safety).

- A useful strategy for these behavioral exercises is to ask the patient to remember how he or she did these activities prior to the military (e.g., was he or she able to sit anywhere in a restaurant, or go to the store whenever he or she needed to rather than at quiet times), and to attempt to approximate that from now on.

- Go to a busy store (e.g., Wal-Mart) for a specified period of time.

- Stand in front of a window or door at night with the shades down or up and lights on or off (vary this depending on level of fear).

- Drive in the middle lane.

- Sit in the middle of a movie theater, restaurant, and so forth.

- In cases of excessive hypervigilant checking, have the patient limit the number of times he or she checks locks and windows or gets up to investigate noises at night.

SUMMARY

We have detailed in this chapter how to conduct an exposure session, with an emphasis on what to do in the context of danger-based principal targets in adaptive disclosure. To a great extent, the strategies recommended are identical to exposure therapy procedures. In addition to an emotion-focused retelling of the experience, we recommend that therapists be very active participant–observers and at times be directive, to help the patient stay with painful content and articulate a narrative about the meaning and implication of the experience (and the experience of disclosing the event). In the case of life-threatening, danger-based events, the change agents entail extinction of conditioned fear (within and between session reductions in the SUDS) and a reduction in constructions of incompetence, dyscontrol, weakness, and self-criticism in the context of postexposure dialogues about the meaning and implication of the event. In the next chapter, we turn to loss and moral injury events. For these experiences, the exposure component remains the same for the most part, but this aspect of the therapy is seen as necessary but not sufficient to promote change.

CHAPTER 8

Breakout Components
for Loss and Moral Injury
Active Treatment Sessions 2 to 7

When service members or veterans are suffering because of a war zone loss or a morally injurious experience, therapists need to augment treatment with what we call *breakout component* sessions. For these patients, raw retelling and discussion of the meaning and implication of the experience are necessary but not sufficient. In adaptive disclosure, we assume that patients need to be exposed to corrective experiences that counter core beliefs about blame, being unforgiven and unforgiveable, and the need to suffer.

In most cases, the principal harm is identified at the outset of therapy. It may also happen that during subsequent exposure sessions the therapist may determine that one of these harms is central to the case. This means that the therapist has learned, or perhaps unearthed sufficient content about the experience, to guide the first and subsequent breakout components. This chapter prepares the therapist to shift to a breakout component, the experiential technique, after the postexposure dialogue in Sessions 2–7.

To reiterate, for service members and veterans who endorse loss or moral injury as their principal harm, the exposure component is designed to iteratively uncover and process specific details or meanings and to create a poignant, charged, and focal emotional state entering the breakout component. In effect, the exposure opens up wounds, with little healing or corrective elements for these types of harms. The shift to the experiential strategies described below provides access to corrective experience and new meanings. The question that should guide therapists' work during the breakout component is: *What does the service member or veteran need to process and do in order to heal from loss or moral injury?*

PREPARING THE SERVICE MEMBER OR VETERAN FOR THE BREAKOUT COMPONENT

The service member or veteran will be asked to transition from the exposure component into having a hypothetical conversation with either the person who has been lost or a forgiving and compassionate moral figure (selected by the service member or veteran prior to Session 2), depending on the breakout component used. If the patient is having difficulty understanding the task, the therapist can spend a few minutes modeling the technique. Well prior to engaging in the breakout component (ideally during Session 1, or at the beginning of Session 2), therapists need to prepare the service member or veteran for the experience by explaining what he or she will be asked to do and how this will help in gaining a different perspective on the incident. The therapist should cover the following points:

> "At some point during the exposure process, I will ask you to shift to having a hypothetical conversation with another person. This is a hypothetical situation; it is not something that necessarily could or will happen. It is an experiment in 'stepping outside of the ordinary' and is distinct from actually engaging in the conversation outside the therapy room. This shift will help you gain a different perspective on your experience and get some 'feedback' from someone who knows you well and cares a great deal about you. The feedback will come from things you realize that person would say or offer, and you will be saying these things aloud and assuming the role of that person in real time."

BREAKOUT COMPONENT FOR LOSS
Prolonged Grief Problems

The death of an important attachment figure or loved one can trigger prolonged grief disorder (PGD; Prigerson et al., 2009), sometimes referred to as "complicated grief" (CG). Formal assessment of PGD is not a requirement for adaptive disclosure; however, clinicians should be aware of the unique phenomenology of PGD, so that they can hypothesize ways of helping their service member or veteran heal from war zone loss. Symptoms of PGD are distinguishable from normal, uncomplicated grief, bereavement-related depression and anxiety symptoms, and PTSD (e.g., Barnes, Dickstein, Maguen, Neria, & Litz, 2012; Boelen & van den Bout, 2005; Bonanno et al., 2002; Prigerson et al., 1995, 1996). Individuals with PGD have been shown to have heightened levels of suicidal thinking and behaviors, poor sleep, reduced quality of life, impaired social functioning, more health complaints, and more days of work missed compared to those without syndromal-level PGD (Boelen & Prigerson, 2007; Bonanno, Moskowitz, Papa, & Folkman, 2005; Chen et al., 1999; Lannen, Wolfe, Prigerson, Onelov, & Kreicbergs, 2008; Latham & Prigerson, 2004; Lichtenthal et al., 2011; Prigerson et al., 1995, 1996, 1997, 2009). For those interested in using PGD in their clinical practice, consensus criteria for PGD have been validated (Prigerson et al., 2009) and will be used in the *International Classification of Diseases* (ICD-11; Maercker et al., 2013).

Prolonged grief problems are more likely to arise when the deceased person is an important attachment figure and especially when the loss is violent and unexpected (Prigerson et al., 2009). *These factors are fundamental to war zone loss.* The complicated bereavement process entails psychological, behavioral, and social disengagement from the present in favor of yearning for the deceased and focusing on the past. Also characteristic of CG are symptoms of anhedonia, guilt about living, and dysphoria, all of which can negatively impact social relationships that are important to recovering from loss. In addition, many bereaved individuals avoid engaging in pleasurable activities because of guilt or concern about exacerbating grief reactions. Consequently, ongoing focal harms from military loss interfere with service members' and veterans' capacity to create and maintain meaningful and supportive relationships and receive mood-enhancing positive reinforcement (e.g., wellness and leisure activities).

Healing from Loss

Specialized evidence-based psychotherapies for PGD (e.g., Shear et al., 2005) encompass two broad categories of change agents: processing the loss with exposure-based experiential strategies and redressing obstacles to positive interpersonal relationships. The exposure-based treatment for entrenched PGD assumes that emotional loss process-ing is required to facilitate impeded grief. Exposure reduces grief, by helping the service member or veteran to relive therapeutically the death scene, and avoidance, by promoting positive experiences in situ-ations the bereaved service member or veteran is avoiding as a result of aversive feelings (intense dread, sadness, guilt). Therapies for PGD designed to redress detachment and disengagement are based on the notion that PGD is caused by the loss of the central focus of one's attach-ment and maintained by the bereaved person's inability to develop and use meaningful interactions with others (Boelen, Van Den Hout, & Van Den Bout, 2006; Shear et al., 2005; Stroebe, Schut, & Boerner, 2010). Such therapies reduce grief by promoting secure alternative attachments to others and emotional reengagement.

In adaptive disclosure, we borrow and extend these intervention strategies. In the context of war-related loss, as we have argued, service members and veterans cannot recover from loss if they only process memories of the loss (exposure component). We assume that service members and veterans who have healed from haunting and guilt-induc-ing war-related loss have done so because they have unburdened them-selves by disclosing the meaning and implication of the experience to others they trust and respect (e.g., peers, family members, and leaders). Furthermore, we assume that these trusted and caring individuals have shared corrective feedback and advice. It is ostensibly this type of posi-tive, hopeful, caring, and corrective advice and feedback that we are try-ing to promote in the loss-related breakout component. In theory, such feedback could come from a trusted therapist, or a loved-one might be invited to therapy sessions. Instead, we go right to the source—the per-son who reciprocated love and devotion—by seeking feedback from the lost attachment figure. This unique change agent depends on the fol-lowing two assumptions: (1) that the dead service member cared deeply about the survivor, would not want him or her to suffer, and would want the best for him or her; and (2) that the surviving service member or vet-eran is capable of voicing these unburdening and hopeful prescriptions.

In adaptive disclosure, we also assume that lasting recovery from consuming war zone loss requires reengagement and reattachment *in vivo* over the life course. Consequently, homework assignments after the loss-related breakout component focus primarily on promoting corrective experiences with self-care and building attachment sys-tems and relational repertoires. Anything is fair game if it promotes reengagement in pleasurable activities, reattachment and forming new attachments, and self-care.

Themes and Dynamics Unique to War Zone Loss

What follows are some observations about grief to focus the therapist's attention and provide a basis for understanding some of the high-probability conflicts that service members and veterans experience related to war zone loss, with suggestions about how to organize the loss-related breakout component.

Responsibility

If a service member or veteran is realistically responsible for the death or injury of a service member, albeit unintentionally (e.g., through a "friendly fire" mistake), grieving the loss requires first forgiving oneself. Self-condemnation can be a sizable obstacle to healing from loss. Another less toxic but much more common form of responsibility for a loss comes from the very nature of the bond that service members have with each other in combat settings, where their lives are literally in each other's hands. In many ways, the relationship that service members and veterans have with one another resembles a parent–child relationship more than it resembles other relationships between adults. Just like a parent caring for a child, every service member in combat feels a personal and immutable responsibility for the survival and safety of the others in his or her unit.

Although service members may never have spoken aloud their commitment to each other's safety, they feel deeply this personal responsibility for each other, and they tend to react with intense feelings of personal failure and guilt for betraying a trust when one of them is lost, *no matter how*. Service members or veterans who are in positions of real responsibility for others, such as unit leaders, may experience survival guilt even more acutely, although they may be less likely to admit this to anyone. This situation gives rise to grief greatly complicated by guilt, and successful navigation of loss depends upon self-forgiveness.

Loss as Trauma

Events are traumatic when they are too intense to be processed successfully and the implications for how one thinks about one's self, other people, and the world are intolerable or ill-suited for optimal functioning. Events can also become unmanageable when the cumulative load on the individual is too great, and he or she becomes worn down and depleted. A relatively "normal" loss can become traumatic, because it afflicts a weakened individual and stands in for all the losses that have preceded it. Thus, even relatively straightforward grief and loss can be traumatic as a function of the intensity and the meanings it holds.

Incomplete Processing

Attachments to peers and leaders in battle are intensely powerful and important. Unit members validate each other's experience, provide respite from the boredom and periodic hell of war, are protective and supportive, and help maintain humanity. Loss of these attachments is profound, challenging beliefs about invulnerability and making service members and veterans feel less safe and grounded. Grief can make a service member lay low, withdraw from other supports, or fail to create new ones. Loss can also create more sensitivity than is desired; intense feelings of grief are incompatible with the warrior identity of feeling strong, invulnerable, focused, optimistic, and powerful. Sometimes grief is hard to manage simply because there is too much of it to process appropriately. There are no social conventions that adequately facilitate the assimilation and accommodation of the onslaught of the senseless loss and destruction that is characteristic of war. Grief after combat losses can be so overwhelming and disorganizing that the only way to manage it is to banish it from awareness in any form.

Almost by definition, and whether or not it is their primary harm, service members or veterans arguably will suffer from incompletely processed grief. In a war zone, there is no time, place, or social structure in which to adequately process grief. Although there are rituals, ceremonies, and such, complete or thorough processing is not likely. The vulnerability that attends grief is a dangerous emotion in theater, and the questions that loss raises are potentially threatening. Grieving and memorializing are safer after return from a combat zone, but the symptoms of prolonged grief, especially initial numbness to emotions and avoidance of memories, can quickly be supplanted with the distraction of preparing for the next deployment, and needing to stay "focused" and to keep one's "edge" for the future.

The case must be made that although it is understandable that sadness and grief would be avoided in theater, for service members, being stateside offers an opportunity to do the work that could not be done then, to honor the dead person, and to figure out how to carry on. Helping service members grieve and process loss is an important role of unit leaders, such as battalion commanders, as well as chaplains. It may be helpful in working with grieving service members or veterans to inquire about how the losses were addressed in the unit and what was done to honor the fallen.

Self-Identity

How we understand our "self" is based in part on how we experience ourselves in relation to others, and this reality is particularly heightened in war. The lost person may represent a part of self, or an experience, that is not readily transferred to or easily shared with another person, making the loss particularly intense. The permanent absence of an important person, particularly someone you care for, threatens all the parts of self that are anchored in the connection with that person. This attachment among service members is akin to the relationship twins have with each other, or how children or adolescents relate with their "best friends" as extensions of the self. Twin-like relationships are common among service members because of the dangers they share and the responsibility they have for each other. In the mind of a twin, the continued existence of his or her mirror image in the world may seem like a prerequisite for his or her own continued existence. In a magical way, the twin might say to him- or herself, "I will be OK as long as my twin is OK." For a service member or veteran, this would translate to "I will be OK as long as my buddy is OK." When that buddy dies, the surviving service member's identity may be significantly threatened.

Guilt

It is hard for many people to feel badly without thinking that they are bad or that they have done something bad. This is particularly true in a military culture, which inculcates the values of agency, power, self-efficacy, and looking out for unit members. Anytime a buddy is lost, there is likely to be a sense that one somehow failed to protect. Sometimes this is a fantasy—a defense against the reality of human helplessness—and other times it is a product of hindsight, and there are times when it is true.

Conflicting Feelings

Seeing what abstract concepts, such as "sacrifice," actually look like in the form of a dead friend risks raising questions about the legitimacy of authority, the war, and the value of the enormous sacrifices being made. These are deeply troubling questions in the aftermath of absolute loss, and the conflicting feelings they activate may cause anguish and with-drawal.

Broken Continuity

Witnessing the destruction of life and seeing vibrant people reduced to body parts threatens one's ability to hold onto a sense of meaning and continuity. The threat of nihilism is brought into focus by traumatic loss. Consequently, even though service members prepare themselves throughout their training for death (their own and others'), the real-ity of death when first experienced by a young person in uniform can result in an intolerable glimpse of his or her own mortality. No service member expects to live forever, but deep down, he or she probably does not expect to die either.

Regardless of the ways in which the grief is experienced, the ther-apist must assume that it can be processed and accommodated. It is important to identify the reasons that, to date, grief has been unap-proachable, and to work directly with those reasons. In addition, just as the simple act of approaching painful material facilitates the undo-ing of avoidance and all its negative associated features; also, reengag-ing in the creative work of psychologically transforming the trauma into something livable (i.e., the very act of reconstructing meaning) is a move against the threat of meaninglessness. Losses are a necessary part of life, and those who master grief are always stronger and wiser than those who have yet to do so.

Processing Loss During the Exposure and Postexposure Dialogue

When the main issue seems to be the sheer intensity of the loss, much can be accomplished during the exposure component. Straightforward exposure to the feelings of intense grief with the aim of facilitating emotional processing, and illuminating and reconsidering the implica-tions of the loss, can be therapeutic. During the exposure component, the preparation for exposure should include basic information that nor-malizes intense feelings of loss and acknowledges the difficulty of pro-cessing this information in theater (e.g., there was probably a "firewall" around the particular loss being processed). While it is a legitimate belief that grieving one loss will provoke the revivification of other losses, it is important to delimit the event being processed (see "Expo-sure Therapy Component: Session Overview" in Chapter 7 for sample dialogue to focus the exposure on a single event). To further clarify the focus on the topic of the experiential breakout, the therapist should ask the service member or veteran:

- "What do you imagine is the risk of or barrier to processing the event?"
- "Do you think that for you the event holds meaning other than loss?"

Questions that may be useful during or after the exposure and breakout components (some of which may already have been addressed) include the following:

"What are you most sad about?"

"What are you most troubled by?"

"How do you think this event has changed you?"

"Is there anything that could have been different?"

"What do you think will happen if you let yourself feel the intensity of your grief?"

"Have there been other times when you've lost someone? If so, how is this similar or different? How did you mourn/grieve in the past?"

Sometimes a service member or veteran may be unable to articulate what, other than sadness and anger, afflicts him or her. In these cases, the therapist can suggest possible areas of difficulty based on the available material. For example, sometimes service members or veterans who have experienced significant loss believe that (1) their sadness or anger is dangerous and will undo them and make them lose the self-control they prize; (2) the experience is too personal to share with others; (3) they will be dishonoring their friend by talking about the experience; (4) they can no longer be the person they were and are broken somehow; (5) the mission has lost its purpose and value; (6) authority is corrupted, and their sacrifices are unappreciated; (7) they are to blame for the loss; and (8) life has less meaning.

When horrific imagery attends a loss, it may be helpful to think of horror and loss as interrelated but separate. One does not grieve horrific imagery or feel sad at its loss; one avoids such triggers and cues. On the other hand, one does grieve and miss the person who is gone and may actually be drawn to psychological or behavioral actions that maintain their presence internally (like holding his or her spot in one's life open and unfilled). In these cases, it may make sense to bracket the exposure to the trauma with imagery of the "whole pretrauma person," so that the two issues are being approached in tandem. In other words, service members or veterans would be asked to describe the person in question, who he or she was, what he or she looked like, and what he or she meant to them. With this as the starting point, the therapist can proceed with an exposure to the traumatic event itself. Once the horror is quieter and the meaning of the loss better illuminated, the therapist can go back to the issue of the lost person and either continue in conversation to rework the relevant meanings or proceed with the breakout component.

Breakout Procedures for Loss

In adaptive disclosure, the therapeutic vehicle to generate hypothesized corrective elements is a conversation with the deceased person. This approach, which is somewhat analogous to the *empty chair* technique in Gestalt therapy, is a useful way of activating other aspects of self that may be helpful and less punitive. It also facilitates the corrective information coming from within the service member or veteran, which will foster mastery and make the potential cognitive shift more compelling. It can be particularly helpful when loss and guilt are entangled, as they often are.

The therapist should incorporate the following sequential steps. First, prior to engaging in the breakout component, the therapist should reiterate the points described in an earlier section of this chapter, "Preparing the Service member or Veteran for the Breakout Component." Second, the therapist should ask the service member or veteran to close his or her eyes and bring up the memory of the lost person when he or she was alive and well, and describe him or her fully. This is done to disclose and process the lost person and to underscore his or her value and potency.

Third, the therapist should instruct the service member or veteran to have a conversation with the deceased person, in real time (right now). This occurs in two phases. In the first phase of this imaginary real-time dialogue, the service member or veteran needs to share the raw details of how the loss is affecting him or her. This should have the flavor of an emotional and very real confession of how the patient feels haunted, ruined, guilty, and incapable of having a good and happy life. It is critical not to allow the service member or veteran to be superficial and disengaged. The therapist needs to be very directive to ensure that the experience is as dramatic, emotional, and powerful as possible. Some prompts that can be used include the following:

> "Now, I want you to go back to the image of [person who died]. This time, I want you to have an actual conversation with him (or her). What would you like to tell him (or her), here, now?"

> "I know he or she is gone, but take this chance to talk to him (or her) and make it real."

> If the service member or veteran gets stuck, the therapist should guide him or her by suggesting: "Why don't you start with what you remember from when he or she was alive? Why don't you talk a bit about how much you miss him, how sorry you are and why?"

After a period of time, the therapist should shift to instructing the service member or veteran to tell the deceased person what has changed in him or her and in his or her behavior since the loss. For example,

- "Tell him (or her) what changed for you after his (or her) death, and tell him (or her) how his (or her) death has affected you. Tell him (or her) how his (or her) death has changed your views of yourself, others, and the world."

- Again, try to get at aspects of how handicapped the person has been since the incident, how he or she has been haunted by the experience, the symptoms he or she has struggled with, and how drastically his life was changed by the experience. For example, the therapist can say: "Tell him (or her) how stuck you are, and be sure to describe [whatever deficits with which service member or veteran has been struggling]."

In the second phase of the dialogue with the lost service member, the goal is to facilitate real-time hypothetical feedback and advice from the dead service member. Most will struggle with this aspect of adaptive disclosure at least to the extent that it is initially awkward and strange to assume the voice of a dead person. If the service member or veteran struggles excessively at any point during this experiential process, the therapist may want to take the voice of either the service member or the service member providing feedback (the deceased), depending on which "voice" is stuck. For example, if the service member or veteran is providing limited feedback from the other figure, the therapist may try to elicit more responses by saying things such as the following:

- "Does this mean I'm bad?"
- "Does this mean I'm crazy?"
- "Does this mean I'm evil?"

Here, the therapist will be taking on the voice of the service member in order to move the conversation to the areas with which the service member or veteran is struggling to verbalize and on which he or she needs feedback. Putting these questions "out there" may help the service member or veteran to consider how the deceased service member or veteran might respond.

The therapist can begin this part of the dialogue by asking the patient to share what the dead person would say to him or her right now, after hearing all of this. For example: "What is he (or she) telling you now, after hearing all you've said?" Allow the service member or veteran time to think about this. The therapist should feel free to introduce content that is forgiveness-related, tailored to the specifics of the case. If the service member's or veteran's responses tend toward the punitive, some shaping prompts might include the following: "Is that honestly what he or she would say? I remember you told me he or she was a great person, who always had your back. What would having your back look like now?"

If this approach fails, ask the service member or veteran to reverse the position, as if he or she were the one who died and was listening to his or her surviving buddy talk about how his or her death was affecting the survivor's life. What would he or she want for the buddy if the situation were reversed? This, we hope, activates forgiveness-oriented themes that the therapist can then extend and emphasize. Ideally, forgiveness themes can emerge, or be coached to emerge, from one of the preceding strategies. Statements that might be inserted when patients are reluctant to do so include the following:

"He (or she) wants you to carry on."

"He (or she) wants what's best for you. What would that look like?"

"There's no doubt that he (or she) wants you to live the fullest life possible."

"This wasn't your fault" (but only if that is true and there is some chance the service member or veteran will agree).

"Even though you didn't do anything wrong, he (or she) forgives you."

"Yes, you screwed up. But, he (or she) believes that even good men (or women) make mistakes. He (or she) forgives you and wants you to claim your life and live it fully *for the both of you.*"

In addressing what the event might come to mean, it is always best if the adaptive meaning can be elicited directly from the service member or veteran, or by his or her recalling what the dead person would say. But if an adaptive construction is not forthcoming, the therapist should be directive, insert the dialogue, and intervene in the meaning-making process directly, making the case for a perspective on the event that he or she feels most likely to be both palatable and adaptive.

This process may be repeated during multiple sessions. After a sufficient amount of processing is done, the therapist should shift to a postbreakout component dialogue about the meaning and implication of the loss and the patient's experience of talking to his or her lost comrade. The therapist starts this by asking the service member or veteran to open his or her eyes and return to the here and now. Then, it is helpful to elicit feedback about his or her experience of what just happened. For example, therapist can ask questions such as the following:

- "What was that like for you?"
- "What are you going to take from this?"

After this, the goal is to have the service member or veteran accommodate the loss by trusting and taking to heart what the dead service member "said to him or her." If the dialogue's meaning and implication of loss fail to have an impact, the conversation needs to be about what drives the resistance (e.g., feeling guilty or undeserving). Further discussion of the postbreakout component dialogue follows in the later section, "Ending the Loss-Related Breakout Component and Session."

Maximizing the Experiential Process and Other Techniques to Use for Loss

There are several things the therapist can do to maximize the experiential process, such as being flexible and willing to try out a few different topics during the loss experiential dialogue if the first topic does not work (e.g., see numbered items on page 114), facilitating imaginal conversations with other individuals besides the lost friend if that does not initially work, and being willing to take on different roles (i.e., being the service member vs. being the friend). Basically, any loss-related topic with which the service member is struggling can be employed during the imaginal conversation. The choice of topics to be used in an experiential dialogue should be based on what the service member or veteran is bringing in that day in relation to the loss, and what is most pressing for the service member or veteran to talk about. Additionally, therapists frequently find that the patient is dealing with more than one distressing theme; therefore, they should be flexible in choosing topics to be confessed and discussed with the dead person, both within and across sessions.

Case Example with Loss

A 29-year-old Gunnery Sergeant who served in Iraq presents with significant PTSD and depression after seeing his best friend "blown to pieces" after hitting an IED. A key part of the trauma is that he chose to take his men in one direction to look for IEDs and told his best friend to take his men in the opposite direction to look for IEDs. As a result, the veteran expressed a great deal of survivor guilt and grief. Possible topics to explore in the experiential dialogue with the lost service member include the following:

> The standard first topic: "What would you want to tell him (or her)? Tell him (or her) what's changed since his (or her) death and how his (or her) death has affected you and your views of yourself, the world, and others. What would he (or she) say back to you?"
>
> If numbing and social withdrawal are prominent: "Talk to him (or her) about how and why your sadness has shifted to numbness and how you have withdrawn from people you care about. Tell him (or her) about your fear of getting close to others now as a result of losing him (or her). Tell him (or her) about the guilt you feel over making new friends. Tell him (or her) what that is like for you and how it is getting in the way of moving on. Tell him (or her) also how the loss has impacted your current relationships. What would he (or she) say about that? What would he (or she) want for you in the future, and how would he (or she) tell you to work through this?"
>
> If guilt about not grieving in theater is prominent: "What would he

(or she) tell you about why it is so difficult to grieve in theater? How would he (or she) want you to go about grieving today?"

If there is a need to review the connection/bond: "What would you tell him (or her) about how he (or she) impacted you? How did he (or she) change you as a service member or veteran? As a person? And what would he (or she) say about how you impacted him?"

If there is a need to say good-bye and honor the lost service member or veteran: "I want you to have a conversation with him (or her) in which you say good-bye. What do you need to say right now? Tell him (or her) about the good memories you want to hold onto of your times together. Tell him (or her) of the image you are going to try to remember of him, rather than that last image you have of him (or her). Tell him (or her) about how you are going to go on to honor him (or her) now. What would he (or she) say to all of this? What would he (or she) want for you moving on?"

If rank is an issue: "What would he (or she) say to you about the challenges a Sergeant, Staff Sergeant, and so forth, faces by grieving in theater? What about being a senior service member or veteran leader (senior noncommissioned officer [NCO]) in theater makes loss more difficult? What are the extra responsibilities you face as a senior leader in theater?"

If Military Operational Specialty (MOS) is a key issue: "What would you say about why it is so difficult to be an infantryman, sniper, mechanic, corpsman, gunner, and so forth? How does this affect your ability to grieve in theater?"

Case Example with Both Loss and Betrayal-Based Moral Injury

A 22-year-old Marine Corporal serving as a sniper in Afghanistan presents with symptoms of PTSD. The Marine's primary trauma involves seeing his best friend blown up in front of him after stepping on an IED. After witnessing this, the Marine then has to engage in a recovery mission, picking up all of the pieces of his dead friend and bagging them. While he presents with a tremendous amount of grief, he also presents with significant anger and a sense of disillusionment as a result of how his friend died. He is extremely angry with his commanders, who sent his unit out on what is perceived to be an unnecessary mission that resulted in the death of his friend (a betrayal-related moral injury). In this case, the choice point is whether to focus on anger as a result of moral injury/disillusionment or to promote loss processing. This service member's anger is so strong that it needs to be processed before any grief work can be done. However, for other service members or veterans, the grief may be so heavy that they have to process it before they can look at the anger.

Possible topics to broach during the loss breakout component in this case (in addition to the grief/loss topics noted earlier) include the following:

> Using the friend to share disillusionment: "Tell your friend about how angry you are about your command. How is this anger getting in the way of your life today? What would he (or she) say back to you about why your commander may have made these choices? What advice does he (or she) have for you? Would he (or she) want this to ruin your life? What would he (or she) want for you?"

> Talking to the leader who betrayed the trust: "I want you to imagine talking to your commander about this event. What do you want to say to him (or her)? Tell him (or her) about how this event is impacting your life. What do you think he (or she) would say to you? What would his (or her) rationale be for the decisions he (or she) made? What could he (or she) say back to you that would make things better? What are you wanting or needing to hear from him (or her)? What if you never hear this from him (or her)?"

Possible Homework Assignments for Loss

As stated, a primary goal in assigning homework assignments is to get the service member or veteran to try to reengage in pleasurable activities and reattach with others. The more the patient engages positively with others, the more opportunities he or she will have to be exposed to corrective information about the loss and to accommodate the messages he or she is hearing (we hope) during the loss-related breakout component. And the more the service member or veteran tries to engage in pleasurable activities, either his or her mood will improve or self-handicapping obstacles that will be revealed can be used as grist for the mill in adaptive disclosure. Consequently, homework should promote positive and secure alternative attachments to others, emotional reengagement, and engagement in positive and reinforcing leisure and wellness activities.

The therapist should ask the service member or veteran two broad sets of questions to guide the selection of homework assignments to foster reengagement and reattachment:

1. "What types of pleasurable or healthy activities are you keeping yourself from doing since the loss of your friend?"
2. "Of those who care about you in your life, who are you not spending quality time with?"

These are starting places in a collaborative dialogue about homework designed to generate a hierarchy of things to do and people to be with, from the most doable to the most difficult and threatening. This process is similar to *activities planning* and *behavioral activation* strategies that have been shown to be helpful in the treatment of depression and prolonged grief (see Cuijpers, Van Straten, & Warmerdam, 2007). The goal is to work with the patient and select an item in the hierarchy to do during the week. The experience should be discussed at the start of the next meeting. Each time, the therapist should evaluate and discuss challenges; obstacles; lessons learned; and changes in mood, constructions, and meanings related to loss.

Another homework area that may help a service member or veteran who is experiencing prolonged grief problems entails doing things that honor the fallen service member. The goal is to facilitate exposure to corrective experiences in the grieving process by honoring the memory of those who have died. As is the case with all homework assignments, this should start with a brainstorming dialogue with the patient, in which the therapist asks, "What do you think might be helpful to do?" Other questions that may be useful to ask are as follows:

"Are there new challenges you might attempt or activities you might devote specifically to the memory of your fallen buddy? Are there life experiences that you might plan partly to honor your fallen buddy?"

"Are there physical ways to memorialize your fallen friend, such as by wearing a bracelet with your buddy's name on it or setting up a website, sign, or placard in your buddy's hometown?"

Since the goal of grieving is to go on with living, without giving up the memory of, or affection for, those who died, any of these celebrations of life in honor of the deceased can be positive and adaptive. And, if nothing else, the act of considering what the fallen buddy would want in the way of a memorial can be constructive, and memorializing him or her can relieve fears of betraying a deceased comrade by getting over feelings of loss too quickly.

Homework assignments can be written, behavioral tasks, or simply issues or thoughts to think about. The therapist should use his or her judgment to determine whether a homework assignment is beneficial, and if so, what assignment naturally fits with the issues with which the service member or veteran is struggling. The therapist must be sure to go over the assignment in the next session. He or she will want to work in a collaborative manner with the service member or veteran to determine what he or she is most willing and able to do for the next week given both patient motivational level and other time commitments he or she may have. For example, the therapist could say any one of the following:

- "What do you think would be useful for you to do before our next session?"
- "What would you be willing to try to work on for next week?"
- "What kind of practice assignment seems doable in the next week?"

Possible written homework options for loss and grief include the following:

- "Think or write about the following:
    - How has losing _____ affected me?
    - How would _____ _____ say I impacted him or her?
    - How did _____ impact me? How have I grown as a person because of _____?
    - How can I honor _____ now and moving forward in my life?
    - What are some of the positive memories I have of _____?"

- "Write a good-bye letter to _____. Include how the loss has changed you, what you'll miss most about the person lost, how you want to remember him or her, and how you will continue to honor him or her."

- How has losing _____ affected my ability to get close to others now?
- What feels so uncomfortable about showing emotions?
- What have I lost due to deployment? What does it mean that I was injured and am now living this way with PTSD (loss of health, identity as a service member or veteran, etc.)?

- "Consider the following possible behavioral options for loss and grief."
  - If the service member or veteran has been avoiding memories of the deceased:
    - Look through pictures of the person or the deployment.
    - Go to the individual's memorial website.
  - Do something to honor lost service member or veteran, such as the following:
    - Wear a personal memorial, such as a bracelet or tattoo.
    - Construct a physical memorial such as a plaque or statue in a public place (e.g., a high school).
    - Donate money or services in memory of the deceased.
    - Organize and lead a celebration of the life the deceased person (e.g., at a church).
    - Write a tribute (or compile a photo collage) to the deceased and offer it to the family as a keepsake for future generations to remember the deceased.
  - Contact buddies who knew the dead service member or veteran and talk about him or her.
  - Volunteer at local military hospitals.
  - Contact the family of the deceased and tell them how much the person meant to you.
  - Share with your partner how losing the person has impacted you and your ability to get close to others.
  - Apologize to the family of the deceased for failing to prevent the death. Consider a symbolic apology, such as a letter that remains unsent, if there is concern that the family will not respond positively.

Ending the Loss-Related Breakout Component and Session

The therapist needs to discuss what the service member or veteran thinks he or she will take from the session. For example, the therapist can ask:

"What do you think you will take from today's session to think
about throughout the week?"

"What really stood out for you?"

In addition, the therapist should normalize temporary elevations
in symptoms. For example:

"I know this was difficult, and more than likely you will continue
to think about it from time to time throughout the week. This
is normal."

"I often find that as service members or veterans start to look at
difficult experiences they've had, they initially experience more
unwanted thoughts about the experience than they had been.
This will go away with time."

The therapist should also assess the service member or veteran at
the end of the session to make sure his or her acute distress has dissipated. If not, discuss what usually makes him or her feel better when
he or she is upset. Encourage these natural coping behaviors or introduce grounding or relaxation techniques prior to ending the session
(see Appendix 2).

BREAKOUT COMPONENT FOR MORAL INJURY

Given the nature of warfare in general, and urban counterinsurgency
guerilla war in particular, it is likely that some service member or veterans will be struggling with moral injury related to their service. Morally injurious experiences are among the most psychologically toxic and
avoided topics (for both therapists and patients). Therapists will need
to be vigilant about the possible presence of these issues and directive to uncover shame-based content. There are two broad categories
of war-related moral injury: perpetration and betrayal-based injuries.

Moral Injury Involving Perpetration

Relevant events and experiences range from the actual perpetration of
acts of unnecessary or capricious violence to perceived acts of commission or omission that violate the service member's or veteran's sense of
honor and duty. Potential morally injurious acts include (but are not
limited to) accidental or intentional killing of noncombatants, torture or
sadistic killing, indiscriminate aggressive behavior or killing (possibly

coupled with suspicion that civilians were killed), mutilation of corpses, sexual assault, failure (real or perceived) to prevent death of comrades, and failure (real or perceived) to prevent death of or atrocity to civilians.

Service members or veterans who have participated in or witnessed such events can sometimes adopt destructive ways of thinking and other negative coping strategies. The first of these is "denial," a self-protective distancing of one's internal view of the world and self-concept from the significance and meaning of potential morally injurious experiences. The maintenance of denial, however, requires increasing amounts of energy, and it often spreads, like a fog, to obscure the significance and meaning of related aspects of life. For example, an individual who remains numb to cope with the memory of committing a violent act toward a child in Iraq may become increasingly numb to the welfare of his or her own children or those of relatives or friends.

Second, once the significance of a potential morally injurious event breaks through self-protective denial, another coping strategy is to allow the incident to overly redefine one's self-concept and identity. Service members or veterans who excessively accommodate to the significance of the incident in this manner may be afflicted with feelings of guilt, shame, disgust, and self-loathing. They are also likely to believe that they are bad people, that everything they tried to be or do in their lives that was good is now negated, and that they deserve an indefinite course of punishment. It is easy to imagine that the increasing suicide rate among combat veterans is related to this maladaptive way of coping with morally injurious events.

The third common maladaptive strategy for coping with moral injury is excessive assimilation of the significance of the event into a preexisting self-schema and worldview. Service members or veterans who use this coping strategy may say to themselves, in effect, "The military is good and just, and I am good and just, so what I did must also be good and just." This can be a slippery slope of negation of wrongdoing, leading to increasingly immoral behavior, if for no other reason than to find the limits of this newly expanded view of right and wrong. It is easy to imagine that misconduct committed by combat veterans is related to this maladaptive strategy for coping with moral injury.

It is important to remember that holding on to the idea of a moral self or a moral code may require that a bad act be judged as such. In other words, maintaining a sense of morality is likely to preclude easy forgiveness of a bad act, and this is not something to be contested. Rather, we want to help the service member or veteran move toward an appreciation of context and the acceptance of an imperfect self. As stated earlier, when discussing belief change, it is unrealistic to expect a complete supplanting of maladaptive beliefs given the brevity of the adaptive disclosure. The goal is to "plant seeds," encourage the consideration of other possible interpretations, and kick-start a process of accommodating transgression without overaccommodating evil and negating any possibility of a positive and good self. This need not entail depicting the service member's or veteran's initial response as entirely incorrect. Instead, the goals of the moral injury breakout component are to challenge extremity and rigidity, and to encourage the awareness that even if a particular act is unequivocally "bad" or "wrong," it is nonetheless possible to move forward and create a life of goodness, value, and making amends. Rather than coping with a morally injurious event by denying it, excessively accommodating to it, or assimilating it into preexisting belief systems, what is needed for adaptive coping is a new synthesis: a new way to view the world and the self that takes into account the reality of the event and its significance, without giving up too much of what was known to be good and just about the self and world prior to the event. As a point of departure from conventional CBT approaches, adaptive disclosure does not assume that anguish, shame, and distress are necessarily caused by distorted thinking. In many instances within the military culture, and especially in the context of the realities and codependencies of units in battle, self-blame or blame of others is not entirely inaccurate. Clinicians also need to know that military training and culture teach service members that their most treasured moral construct, honor, is earned through actions that are just, moral, and ethical, and sacrifices that are noble. Indeed, perceived transgression is particularly anguishing and disruptive because it undermines service members' moral identities by damaging their trust in their sustaining moral values and guiding ideals, or in their own abilities to follow them. In adaptive disclosure, the goal is not necessarily to help the patient challenge the veracity of these conclusions; rather it is to respect and honor where they come from while promoting more adaptive and sensible future possibilities.

In the moral injury breakout component, all acts of moral injury must be examined within two frameworks: *the fulcrum of war* and *the totality of the self.* The purpose of bringing these contexts into the picture is neither to create a relative moral code nor to minimize the service member's or veteran's acts. Rather, it is to locate those acts within the broader reality of both the situation and the person, and in doing so bring these other relevant aspects into contact with the memory, so that the service member or veteran begins to incorporate them. These broader realities facilitate a more nuanced remembrance and integration with the rest of the service member's or veteran's knowledge and life. If the principal harm can be viewed within a fuller understanding of self and time–place, then it is possible to work toward balance, perspective, and proportionality in how it is experienced. Therefore, the moral injury should be examined during the exposure component and the moral injury breakout within the context of the war, as well as the events leading up to it and the service member's moment-to-moment experience of what happened. In addition to bringing the larger war context into the picture, the service member or veteran must be encouraged, cognitively, to draw a circle around the totality of his or her life and self. Within the circle will be the event in question, but it also must include all the more positive parts of self, as well as the possibility of future positive actions. In this way, it becomes possible to maintain a moral universe (as compared to a relativistic one) without allowing one part to shadow unduly or cancel out the rest. Homework exercises (described later in this chapter) are essential to provide exposure to corrective information to reinforce this sense of goodness and to begin the process of repairing by making amends.

Special Considerations for the Therapeutic Relationship

The moral injury breakout component is designed to promote accommodation of new, forgiving, and compassionate information. The connection with and response of the therapist to move against shame, isolation, and interpersonal fear are also critical. Although the latter is operative throughout, nowhere is it more central or more endangered by the nature of the problem than in the moral injury breakout component.

In preparation for working with a service member or veteran who may have engaged in excessive violence, it is important that the therapist imagine, ahead of time and in detail, the range of possible acts of gratuitous violence, and figure out how to tolerate this kind of material while genuinely accepting the service member or veteran. Even in an encounter as brief as this one, the genuine relationship of the therapist to the service member or veteran and the story he or she is telling will be a critical component of how the event comes to be experienced. The therapist will need to model—implicitly and explicitly—acceptance, compassion, and forgiveness.

Any tacit disgust or fear expressed by the therapist, even to elements of the narrative unrelated to the service member's or veteran's role, will be experienced as condemnation. Frozen professionalism and detachment, while understandable, are also not therapeutic responses. Even if the service member or veteran is retelling acts of perpetration, a therapist must find within the story or the person the elements around which true empathic connection can be summoned. The assumption needs to be that regardless of the nature of the transgression, if a service member is experiencing shame and guilt, and seeking treatment for his or her suffering, then the service member has premorbid goodness and a moral core. It is essential that therapists familiarize themselves with some of the horrible things that people do and witness in war. Closely reviewing these kinds of events, while imagining him or herself sitting with the perpetrator, will give the therapist a chance to experience and examine his or her feelings of horror and condemnation without harming an actual patient. This type of preparation should also give the therapist the opportunity to examine his or her feelings of judgment and desire to distance, in order to move into a place where he or she can imagine either committing a similar act or loving someone who has done so.

These preparatory tasks parallel the enormous challenge faced by the service member or veteran within therapy. That is, just like the service member or veteran, the therapist must imagine embracing, with warmth and acceptance, a complex self that contains the capacity for committing evil acts. The therapist's humble consideration of the context of war, as well as his or her experience with trauma work and time in supervision around these issues, should facilitate his or her capacity to remain warm, emotionally present, and empathic.

Just as it is critical for the therapist to be fully emotionally present, it is also critical, and even more difficult, for the service member or veteran to be fully emotionally engaged. The emotions and meanings associated with moral injury involving perpetration are extraordinarily aversive and threatening. Service members or veterans will be motivated to avoid these at all costs. However, deep emotional engagement is central to hot (as opposed to cold or emotionless) emotion-based cognitive processing during the moral injury breakout component. Service members or veterans need to experience thinking and feeling deeply about these issues, or they will bury the content and close themselves off to new perspectives and learning. Approaching these horrifying thoughts and feelings in the presence of an accepting other—within the framework of the unique hell of war and the reality that worthwhile people do terrible things—will activate the beginnings of acceptance, the possibility of growth, and continued movement. Finally, therapists always need to bear in mind that this growth will need to go well beyond their brief time with the service member or veteran.

Moral Injury Involving Betrayal

Betrayal experiences chiefly stem from leaders' behaviors and judgments that are capricious, dangerous, and entail grossly unfair mistreatment. In other words, individuals violated expectations of moral and ethical conduct, with horrific consequences. The betrayal is also likely to be associated with no attendant redress or justice. Consequently, in this form of moral injury, the service member's or veteran's confidence in moral authority and moral structures is shaken, if not obliterated. At various points in adaptive disclosure, the therapist should assess the impact of betrayal. For example, he or she can ask, "Are there things about your experience that you find you cannot forgive others for—either things that superiors, peers, or even the enemy did, or things that they didn't do but should have? Difficulty forgiving others can cause persistent anger and a wish for retribution or revenge. Forgiving others without exacting "justice" through retaliation can be difficult for anyone who has experienced a betrayal, and the consequences of unresolved feelings of betrayal on beliefs about the trustworthiness of peers or figures of authority can be profound. The therapist should explore with the service member or veteran the consequences of carrying such unresolved feelings of betrayal. The goal is to start to understand how the betrayal has affected the service member's or veteran's ability to trust others, believe in institutions, and value ideals such as right and wrong. The therapist can ask the patient to consider the added injustice of the distress and loss of social or occupational functioning caused by someone else's actions or failures to act.

Betrayal-based moral injury leads to anger and overgeneralized irritability, blaming, expectations of injustice, acting-out, revenge fantasies, inability to forgive, and externalizing attributional bias (poor responsibility-taking). For these unique moral injuries, the goal of the breakout component is to express anger and disappointment, unburden feelings and thoughts of being a helpless victim of another's immorality, and accommodate both the immoral behavior of others and the notion of living comfortably in a world where this can happen.

Clinical Stance and Overall Approach to Moral Injury

The overall therapeutic frame for the moral injury breakout component is that through facing and examining seemingly intolerable events and meanings will come the strength and perspective to determine how to go forward and continue to make a positive contribution. In general, service members or veterans have a powerful sense of good and evil.

There are many advantages to a clear and delineated worldview in this regard. However, there is also the probability of black-and-white thinking, which in turn leads people to decide that they are either good or bad. A service member or veteran who has transgressed, or believes he or she has done so, may conclude: *"I am evil, I am worthless, I can never forgive myself, and I don't deserve to live or have a decent life."* Alternatively, the service member may conclude the opposite global and absolute judgments: that they did nothing wrong and all those who suffered at their hands deserved it. The following are descriptions of clinical presentations and issues that need to be addressed directly during the moral injury breakout component.

Guilt and Shame

It is worth taking some time to assess with the service member or veteran the reality basis of his or her sense of culpability. Service members or veterans may feel guilty for not preventing the impossible and for anything that is less than ideal and perfectly heroic behavior. These are not realistic standards, and they should be challenged. It is common for people to exaggerate guilt by overestimating the control they have over conditions. If a comrade died or someone suffered injury, the service member or veteran will often feel that he or she should have prevented it. It can be useful to ask the service member or veteran to explain how it occurred and how it realistically could have been avoided. In these cases, keep an ear open for statements that ignore the facts of the event and suggest that the service member or veteran should have had superhuman ability (e.g., ignoring the speed of events, stress occurring at the time, the extent to which he or she followed operational procedures, being wise in hindsight but expecting him- or herself to see things in advance). These unrealistic expectations need to be challenged directly and repeatedly. In the ideal case, the corrective perspective will come from the service member or veteran as he or she articulates what a loving, forgiving, and compassionate moral authority would say as he or she discloses these rigid ideas about culpability during the moral injury breakout component described below. However, therapists have to be directive, speaking for the moral authority in many instances and for themselves in the post-moral injury breakout dialogue. In this context, the therapist should discuss these ways of thinking in terms of the need to defend against the reality of our limitations, that is, as a defense against helplessness. The acceptance of universal human limits and the willingness to do one's best anyway is a greater strength, one born of maturity, than unrealistic visions of heroism.

In other cases, when culpability is unclear; the therapist and service member or veteran may be unable to come to agreement (presumably with the service member or veteran taking more responsibility); or both the therapist and the service member or veteran may agree that there is indeed culpability. Service members or veterans may, justifiably, use as a frame of reference the reality that while everyone is confronted by the stresses of war, only some people cross the line into truly bad acts. This is true, and it is not worth getting stuck by arguing whether there is moral responsibility. In these cases, the frame becomes, simply, how to face it in such a way as to move forward productively, through experiencing forgiveness and engaging in repair-oriented behaviors.

In adaptive disclosure, the intent is to create an atmosphere in which a forgiving and compassionate moral authority, sometimes through the voice of the patient and other times through the voice of the therapist, asks the service member or veteran to consider his or her condemning conclusions in light of the war experience itself and the stressors leading up to the event. At times, patients may have difficulty coming up with a compassionate moral authority, or another important, salient figure may be more powerful or appropriate. For example, another salient figure might be a subordinate service member, another veteran, or the harmed victim.

War asks people to do and experience things far outside what our moral code prepares us to anticipate and cope with. It is an atypical situation that distorts the normal rules of morality and behavior. Often there is no preparation for the levels of rage, fear, guilt, and grief that often precede an egregious act in combat. Under the pressure of intense emotions, the clarity between right and wrong can be blurred. People often engage in antisocial or bizarre behavior during war, because actions are required that would never occur in peacetime. In war, such behavior is, to a large extent, expected and leads military personnel to adjust their normal rules of moral behavior. In these conditions, service members or veterans may have committed acts about which they feel guilty.

It is also important to facilitate the moral authority (or other salient figure) helping the patient to separate the overall worth of the individual from a particular act. The fact that someone did something bad does not render any other good he or she has done in his or her life null and void, nor does it change who he or she is at the core or who he or she might become over the course of life. The service member or veteran should be asked to consider the totality of his or her life and actions. As homework, it may be helpful to have the service member or veteran write out his or her values and how he or she has carried out these beliefs in positive ways. Sometimes, good people do bad things. A life is made up of many moments and many acts, and through the conversation with the moral authority (described below), the patient and therapist can make the case that the different parts do not cancel each other out; they simply coexist.

THINKING ABOUT AND PLANNING TO MAKE AMENDS

Particularly in cases of acts of commission, it may be useful to suggest that staying stuck and impaired does not erase or balance out the wrong that occurred. Instead, there are ways to live that move toward decency and goodness, and that are helpful to other people. While it is impossible to "fix" events in the past and, indeed, any focus on literal repair will likely ring hollow, there is the notion of making amends. To "amend" means, literally, to change. "Making amends" means drawing a line between past and present, and in some way changing one's approach to living, in order to move toward the positive and toward better behavior. It is necessary that this process be very concrete and detailed. The therapist should ask the service member or veteran to make a list of who was hurt, how and why, in the service of facilitating a meaningful reckoning of the threatening material and thereby open the way for the therapist to have input into the patient's self-judgments. After this is done, plans for moving forward in part by making amends can be delineated. While there may not always be sufficient time to flesh-out this idea fully, elements may be assigned for homework and a path laid out for future growth and change.

This work must be approached carefully. It does not and should not emanate from within a punishment framework but from an empathic appreciation of the decency that drives the desire to be a good person. Guilt may be understood as a useful attention-getting feeling. It is not a feeling on which to linger or indulge but is instead a call for change, activating the need for some type of corrective action that must be enacted. Be vigilant that this idea of making amends can sometimes also be taken to an extreme; patients can come to feel that they must focus their lives only on activities that will "right their wrong." The idea of righting a wrong is usually a poor idea, because it is typically not possible (however, if there is real action that can undo something, then by all means explore this). In general, the idea is not to try and fix the past but to draw a firm line around the past and its related associations, thoughts, and feelings, so that the mistakes of the past do not define the present and the future, and so that a preoccupation with the past does not prevent possible future good.

RELIGIOUS BELIEFS

It is helpful to know the service member or veteran's religious beliefs/ traditions. While candid disclosure to a therapist and reception of an empathic and nonjudgmental response can be enormously helpful, it may be that a discussion with *an actual moral authority figure* is warranted. This can be suggested as homework or as a future step if it seems appropriate and helpful. The hope is that faith, communion with, and empathy from others who share a faith, and messages based on "good" theology—centered on love and forgiveness—will help heal moral injuries over time.

Breakout Procedures for Moral Injury

In adaptive disclosure, the therapeutic vehicle to generate hypothesized corrective elements is a conversation with a benevolent moral authority. This approach, which is somewhat analogous to the *empty chair* technique in Gestalt therapy, is a useful way of activating other aspects of self that may be helpful and less punitive. It also facilitates the corrective information within the service member or veteran that will foster mastery and make the potential cognitive shift more compelling. Below, we provide separate, specific instructions for the therapeutic dialogue with the moral authority, one for perpetration-based moral injuries and another for betrayal-based experiences.

Perpetration-Based Moral Injury

Once the presence of moral injury is ascertained, the service member or veteran needs to select a person for whom he or she has great respect and can imagine weighing in as a relevant, generous, forgiving, and compassionate moral authority. After the exposure component (see Chapter 7), the patient is asked to have a conversation in imagination with this moral authority. It may be that the presence of moral injury is only ascertained during or after the standard imaginal exposure procedure, in which case, this step can be carried out immediately after the standard exposure has concluded.

Great care must be taken in setting up and choosing this person.

The requirement is that the service member or veteran think of someone who has always had his or her back and has been and will continue to be in his or her corner, *no matter what*. The individual needs to have his or her best interests at heart and be someone who is respected (parent, teacher, leader, friend, God, etc.). If the patient absolutely cannot think of someone like that, then legitimate and personally meaningful figures in religious or popular culture should be considered.

Once the moral authority is identified, the therapist should incorporate the following steps. First, the therapist should reiterate the points described in the previous section, "Preparing the Service Member or Veteran for the Breakout Component." If modeling the conversational technique is necessary, the therapist can suggest that the service member or veteran close his or her eyes and have a brief conversation (e.g., about a recent conflict with a peer or family member) with a trusted friend.

Next, the therapist should instruct the service member or veteran to have a conversation with the moral authority in real time (right now). This occurs in two phases. In the first phase of this imaginary real-time dialogue, the service member or veteran needs to disclose (confess) the morally injurious experience *to the moral authority*. The service member or veteran should engage in this task with his or her eyes closed and using the present tense. It is critical not to allow the service member or veteran to be superficial and disengaged. The therapist needs to be very directive to ensure that the experience is as dramatic, emotional, and powerful as possible for the service member or veteran. To transition from the postexposure dialogue, the therapist can say:

> "With your eyes closed again, I want you to picture [moral authority figure]."
>
> "Do you have an image of _____? What does he or she look like?"

The therapist should then shift to instructing the service member or veteran to disclose the incident to the moral authority. For example:

> "I want you to tell him (or her) what you did (or failed to do)."
>
> "What do you want to say to him (or her) right now?"

If the service member or veteran gets stuck, the therapist should guide him or her, for example, by saying: "Tell him (or her) how sorry you are that this happened. Tell him (or her) why this happened."

It is important that the patient relive the transgression, knowing that the moral authority is listening and watching, so to speak. *This is the key distinction between the exposure component and the breakout component with respect to reliving the transgression.* As with the exposure component, the therapist should have the patient relive all the details and share any and all raw thoughts and feelings about the event. Also, he or she should ask the patient to share, in the here and now, what the event means about him or her as a human being, given that he or she did (or did not) do something. In other words, the patient needs to unearth all the raw thoughts, meanings, and feelings, and implications of the transgression. This is very much akin to a frank emotional confession, in this case, to a secular moral authority.

It is particularly important to instruct the service member or veteran to tell the moral authority figure what has changed in him or her and in his or her behavior since the event. For example:

> "Tell him (or her) what changed for you since this happened, and tell him how this event has affected you."

Here, the aim is to try to get at aspects of how handicapped the service member or veteran has been since the incident, how he or she has been haunted by the experience, the symptoms with which he or she has struggled, and how drastically his or her life was changed by the experience. For example, the therapist can say:

> "Tell him (or her) how stuck you are. Tell him (or her) how undeserving you feel of happiness."

The second phase of the dialogue with the moral authority is hearing what the moral authority has to say about what he or she just heard—to get real-time therapeutic feedback. The patient's job is to speak with the voice of the moral authority in real time. This can be prompted by asking the patient the following questions:

> "What does _____ think about what you just shared with him (or her)?"
>
> "What does he or she think about all of this?"
>
> "What does he or she want to tell you?"
>
> "What advice does _____ want to give you?"

In this phase of the dialogue, the therapist should try to ensure that the moral authority is, to a degree, disappointed and realistically surprised, if not shocked, by what he or she just heard. The assumption here is that a loved one would be surprised, because he or she typically would not be aware of any propensity or risk for moral transgression, nor would he or she be aware of the vagaries of war.

Once the spontaneous spoken feedback is exhausted, the therapist should transition to ensuring that the moral authority speaks with an understanding, compassionate, and forgiving voice. Some questions to trigger or prompt follow:

"Ask _____ whether he (or she) could forgive you."

"Ask _____ whether he (or she) still loves you."

"Does _____ think that you should only suffer the rest of your life as a result of this?"

"Tell him (or her) what you would like to do to make amends."

Again, if the service member or veteran struggles at any point during the experiential process, the therapist needs to take the voice of either the service member/veteran, or the moral authority, depending on which "voice" is stuck. For example, if the service member or veteran is saying too little to the moral figure, the therapist may say things like the following:

"Does this mean I'm bad?"

"Does this mean I'm crazy?"

"Does this mean I'm evil?"

Here, the therapist will be taking on the voice of the service member or veteran in order to move the conversation to the areas that he or she is struggling to verbalize and on which he or she needs feedback. Putting these questions "out there" may help the service member or veteran to consider what the moral authority figure might say to him or her.

The therapist can introduce content that is compassionate, understanding, and forgiveness-related, tailored to the specifics of the case, such as the following:

"He (or she) wants you to carry on."

"He (or she) wants what's best for you."

· "There's no doubt that he (or she) would want you to live the fullest life possible."

"He (or she) forgives you."

"He (or she) understands why this happened, and wants you to know you are forgiven."

This process may be repeated during multiple sessions. After a sufficient amount of processing is done, the therapist should shift to a postbreakout component dialogue about the meaning and implication of the incident and the patient's experience of talking to the moral authority. The therapist can start by asking the service member or veteran to open his or her eyes and return to the here and now. Then, it will be helpful to elicit feedback about his or her experience of what just happened. For example, the therapist can ask the following questions:

"What was that like for you?"

"What are you going to take from this?"

After this, the goal is to have the service member or veteran accommodate the incident by trusting and taking to heart what the moral authority "said to him or her." If the meaning and implication of the incident are not impacted by the dialogue, the conversation needs to be about what drives the resistance (e.g., feeling guilty or undeserving). Further discussion of the postbreakout component dialogue follows in the section "Ending the Moral Injury Breakout Component and Session."

Betrayal-Based Moral Injury

In the case of betrayal-based moral injury, the dialogue with a wise, caring, compassionate, and respected person is similar in structure to the previous dialogue, but the content focuses on the report of the violation of another (e.g., a leader) and the impact and implications of the experience for the service member or veteran (angry all the time, withdrawn, uncaring, loss of moral compass, etc.). This is followed by constructive and corrective feedback from the person (in imagination) who, in theory, would not only be similarly outraged by the abhorrent and morally corrupt action but also invested in this experience not ruining the service member's or veteran's life. The therapist should guide the dialogue, if necessary, so that healing and corrective themes are expressed. In terms of betrayal, a caring, wise, and compassionate friend or mentor would not want the experience to turn a positive person into a dark and angry service member or veteran, family member, parent, or citizen.

Alternative Strategies

As was the case with the loss-related breakout component, therapists should use their discretion about incorporating any number of moral injury-related themes or angles or replacements for the moral authority chosen by the patient. The following are case-based examples with different topics to try.

PERPETRATION-BASED MORAL INJURY CASE EXAMPLE

A 21-year-old Marine Lance Corporal who served as an infantryman in Afghanistan presents with significant PTSD. He is particularly struggling with the numerous killings he engaged, as well as his feelings of excitement, pride, and happiness at the time of the killings. Varied options for topics to address with the moral authority include the following:

> The standard default dialogue: "What would you want to tell him (or her)? Tell him (or her) how sorry you are. Tell him (or her) why you did what you did. Tell him (or her) what you will do to make amends. Tell him (or her) what's changed since this event. Tell him (or her) how stuck you've been. What does he or she want to tell you now that he or she has heard of all this?"

> Military rank and role issues: "What do you need to tell him (or her) about why it is so difficult to be an infantryman, sniper, mechanic, corpsman, gunner, senior enlisted (etc.)? How did this impact how you acted out there?"

> Contextualizing war, engagements, or battle: "After listening with an open heart about what you just said, what would _____ say to you about what about war causes service members to think, feel, and do things they would not anticipate doing? What would he or she say to you about the initial invasion, serving in Afghanistan, the battle of Fallujah, this particular firefight that caused you to act the way you did? What would he or she say to you about this war that is particularly difficult and contributed to how you acted and felt?"

Using a Person about Whom the Service Member or Veteran Feels Protective as the Moral Authority

If, for whatever reason, it appears that a conversation with a moral authority is too much of a stretch for the service member or veteran, ask him (or her) to think of someone toward whom he or she feels protective (e.g., a junior service member or veteran, or a younger brother). In this context, the process entails asking the service member or veteran to mentor this person: He or she becomes the person who violated the moral standard and is self-damning. In this case, the younger person is asking for guidance from someone more mature. The service member or veteran is asked to take on the role of this person who shares what he or she did (what the service member or veteran did); they are the one confessing the actions that he or she (the service member or veteran in treatment) has committed or failed to do, and to listen to him describe how this is affecting the young person. In this context, this is like an imaginary role-reversal. The following are some examples:

> Military operational specialty/rank: "What would you say to a junior service member or veteran/boot/younger corpsman/and so forth about why it is so difficult to be an infantryman, sniper, mechanic, corpsman, gunner, senior enlisted, and so forth in theater? What are the special difficulties you face out there? How did this impact how he or she may have acted out there?"

> Context of war, difficulties of this war, or difficulties of a given battle: "What would you say to him (or her) about the aspects of war that cause men or women to think, feel, and do things they would not anticipate doing? What would you say to him (or her) about the initial invasion, serving in Afghanistan, the battle of Fallujah, or this particular firefight that caused him to act the way he or she did? What would you say to him (or her) about this war that is particularly difficult and contributed to how he or she acted and felt?"

Shame about a Highly Charged and Personal Killing

In this context, it may be useful to have the service member or veteran to imagine talking *to the person he or she killed*. Here the therapist would guide a highly charged imaginary dialogue with the victim. The therapist could say:

"I want you to describe the man/woman/child (or their family members) you killed. What did he or she (or they) look like before and after (if known)? I want you to talk to him (or her, or them). What do you want to say? What would be important about the situation for him or her (or them) to know? Tell him or her (or them) how his or her (or their) death has impacted you. How has it changed you? Tell him or her (or them) how sorry you are. Tell him or her (or them) what you are doing in your life to make amends. What does he or she (or they) say back to you? What would you like him or her (or them) to say?"

Possible Homework Assignments for Moral Injury

Homework assignments can be written, action-oriented/behavioral, or simply things to think about in between sessions. Decisions about homework should always be collaborative and, ideally, come chiefly from the service member or veteran. Nevertheless, the therapist should use his or her judgment to determine whether a homework assignment would be beneficial, and if so, what assignment would naturally fit well with issues with which the service member or veteran is struggling. The therapist will want to make sure to go over the assignment in the next session, either in the beginning or during the processing phase of the session. To work collaboratively, the therapist can initiate a dialogue about homework with questions such as the following:

"What do you think would be useful for you to do before our next session?"

"What would you be willing to try to work on for next week?"

"What kind of practice assignment seems doable for you to work on in the next week?"

Possible Written Options or Thought Experiments for Moral Injury

The patient can think or write about the following:

• What makes people do things in war that they would not normally do (or would not have anticipated doing)?

• What were some of the factors going on just prior to this incident that may have contributed to me (or others) acting this way?

- What are the costs–benefits of feeling guilt, anger, or shame? What does my future look like if I continue to hold onto all of these feelings? What might it look like if I started to accept and move past these experiences?

- "Write about what you've gained from and will take from your time in the military, and what you'll be happy to leave behind."

- "Write about forgiveness of self and others: What about your deployment experiences (if anything) are you having a hard time forgiving yourself for? Forgiving others for? What are things about which you are self-critical or self-condemning? What are things for which you criticize/condemn others?"

- "Write about compassion for self and others: The Dalai Lama (the head of Tibetan Buddhism) defines compassion as 'a sensitivity to the suffering of self and others with a deep wish and commitment to relieve the suffering' (i.e., being able to show sympathy for yourself or others). What does compassion mean to you, and do you think you could be compassionate and forgiving of yourself and others? If you don't think you could ever be compassionate and forgiving of yourself or others, why?"

- "Write a plan of intention and motivation to be compassionate and forgiving of self and others."

- "What are some of the things for which you are having a hard time forgiving yourself or others?"

- "Brainstorm about the things you could do in order to start forgiving yourself or others. This could be actual physical behaviors you do, or simply changing the way you think about things. Brainstorming means allowing yourself to think of as many different solutions as possible, even if they don't seem realistic. Later we'll go through these things and I can help you judge what is best to consider actually doing."

- "Think about specific steps you can take this week to start forgiving yourself or someone else."

- "Think about specific steps you can take over the next few months to start forgiving yourself or someone else."

Homework Considerations for Perpetration-Based Moral Injury

The patient can think or write about the following:

Totality of self: "List things you are proud of in your life (e.g., things about yourself; positive things you've done) and things you are less proud of, especially things that show your goodness and worthiness, focusing particularly on as many things you are proud of as possible. Consider things that happened before, during, and after military service."

"Write a letter to _____ (victim). What would you want to say to them?"

"Write about what you felt you did particularly well that day, and what you wish you had done differently."

"What does this mean about you as a person that you've done _____?"

"What do you think would happen if you acted in a compassionate way with yourself and forgave yourself? What does the guilt you are experiencing look like on a day-to-day basis? What are the thoughts, feelings, and behaviors you engage in because you are feel guilty? How does holding onto the guilt get in the way of your life? How could your future look if you were able to forgive yourself?"

"Write a letter to yourself from a caring, loving, compassionate moral authority: What does he or she or she think about what you have done? What do they think this means about you as a person? What does he or she or she think about your potential as a person moving forward? What does this person tell you about how you are suffering right now? How does this person express compassion and forgiveness to you?"

"What are steps you will likely be taking over the course of your life to work on forgiving yourself or others?"

"Who are you angry with? What are you most angry about?"

"Write a letter (not to be sent) to the offender, the person who betrayed you. Speak to why you are so angry and bitter. Share how this experience has changed how you feel about yourself as a person and as a service member or veteran. Also, share how this experience has changed how you feel about people in positions of power and authority in the military and in general. However, also in this letter, I want you to try to put yourself in their shoes and imagine all of the possible reasons why the person did what he or she did. Imagine being able to forgive this person and forgive what they did or failed to do. Also, imagine being compassionate about this person and what they did or failed to do. If you were forgiving and compassionate, what would you say in this letter?"

"Write about betrayal: What do you think would happen if you acted in a compassionate way with others and forgave others? How would this impact how you see the event? What does the anger and hurt you are experiencing look like on a day-to-day basis? What are the thoughts, feelings, and behaviors you engage in because you are angry or hurt? How does holding onto the anger and hurt from the incident get in the way of your life? How would your future look if you were able to let go of this anger and hurt?"

"Imagine being assigned as an attorney to represent the person with whom you are angry. How could you make the case for the actions he or she took that day? For example, were there any extenuating circumstances that may have impacted what occurred (consider his or her frame of mind, context of the event, role of others, events outside of his or her control)?"

Possible action-oriented (behavioral) options for perpetration-based moral injury:

Talk about guilt and shame with a trusted person.

Privately apologize to the person who was wronged or wronged person's family, if possible. (Note to therapist: Pursue this cautiously depending on likely response from wronged person— this may need to be symbolic.)

Symbolically (through an unsent letter or role play) explain to either the victim or his or her family the limits of one's culpability (e.g., "I did this, but I did not do that" or "I didn't intend it to happen," or even "I wanted to prevent it from happening but couldn't").

Symbolically "repay the debt" by giving something of value (goods, money, service) to an organization or other social group that can serve as a proxy for the person wronged.

Perform acts of goodness to reinforce a positive self-concept.

Seek out positive restorative experiences or opportunities to make amends when an actual deed cannot be undone (e.g., registering to become an organ donor; giving blood).

If guilt involves children and the therapist feels comfortable that service member or veteran can interact positively with children: Make amends by trying to have a positive impact on a child's life (Big Brother/Big Sister; hospital volunteer; sponsor a remote child by remote, say, one in Africa). Volunteering at a shelter or adopting an animal might be another alternative.

Possible behavioral tasks for betrayal-based moral injury:

Ask for an apology/ask for retribution—this may need to be symbolic.

Forgive.

Seek civil compensation or criminal justice.

Symbolically "defeat" the perpetrator by effectively supporting other victims of similar wrongdoing.

Symbolically "defeat" the perpetrator by working to prevent similar wrongdoing in the future.

Symbolically forgive the perpetrator by showing compassion to other, similar perpetrators.

Ending the Moral Injury Breakout Component and Session

The therapist needs to discuss what the service member or veteran thinks he or she will take from the session. For example, the therapist can ask:

"What do you think you will take from today's session to think about throughout the week?"

"What really stood out for you?"

In addition, the therapist should normalize temporary elevations in symptoms. For example:

- "I know this was difficult, and more than likely you will continue to think about it from time to time throughout the week. This is normal."

- "I often find that as service members or veterans start to look at difficult experiences they've had, they initially experience more unwanted thoughts about the experience than they had been. This will go away with time."

The therapist should also assess the service member or veteran at the end of the session to make sure his or her acute distress has dissipated. If not, discuss what usually makes him or her feel better when he or she is upset. Encourage these natural coping behaviors or introduce grounding or relaxation techniques prior to ending the session (see Appendix 2).

FOR LOSS OR MORAL INJURY: THE BLAME/FORGIVENESS/ AMENDS EXERCISE

It is important for therapists to understand that in the military, the core values and warrior ideals of love and honor are powerful motivators, and the shame that results from the loss of honor is even more powerful (see Chapter 3). Because of the culture and ethos of the military, it is safe to assume that nearly all service members and veterans who have suffered a war zone loss or moral injury are in part haunted by thoughts of personal weakness, failure, responsibility, and self-blame. No psychotherapy can fully eradicate the "what ifs" about personal culpability that drive feelings of guilt over the life course. The goals of adaptive disclosure are to help the service member or veteran construct less rigid and less absolute self-condemning judgments over time and to think of ways to take action to seek or create forgiveness of self or others.

The following exercise is designed to help service members or veterans go through a thought process about blame that can provide opportunities for perspective taking, assess otherwise rigid beliefs about responsibility, and actively consider making amends and seeking forgiveness. This exercise should be used liberally throughout adaptive disclosure. The goal is to help service members and veterans assess the level of their own and others' culpability in a useful way, as well as think about ways to make or seek amends in order to feel more forgiven or forgiving.

First, on a sheet of paper, the service member or veteran names *all* the people, institutions, or things (e.g., one's own stressed-out brain) who might be (or feel) responsible for the loss or morally injurious events. Second, the service member or veteran assigns *percentage of responsibility* to each person or agency on the list, from 0 to 100%, making sure that the total of all culpabilities does not add up to more than 100%. Third, on a scale of 1 to10, the service member or veteran states the degree to which each person or thing on the list *is currently forgiven*. Fourth, the service member or veteran brainstorms about specific methods that he or she could use either to *make* or to *seek amends* to promote forgiveness, and prioritizes them. Then, if appropriate, the therapist helps the service member or veteran make homework plans to do one of these things to make or seek amends. If any item is agreed upon during the week as a homework assignment, it is important to follow up on progress toward completion and rerating levels of forgiveness.

DISCRETION ABOUT REPEATING THE EXPOSURE COMPONENT

The exposure and breakout components share some common features that may be quite repetitive, which may cause frustration. In the context of loss and moral injury, the exposure component is used to discover new material and to process new meanings that may not arise in the context of the "confessional" breakout component but may be processed in a subsequent breakout. However, if the exposure component and dialogue fail to unearth additional salient content or modified meanings and implications across sessions, the therapist may opt to discontinue the exposure component in favor of emphasizing the breakout component for the entire session.

SUMMARY

In this chapter, we have described in detail the specific strategies and techniques pertaining to the loss and moral injury breakout components of adaptive disclosure. These two breakout components distinguish adaptive disclosure from other psychotherapies for war-related PTSD. Because of the novelty of these change agents and therapeutic processes, clinicians should expect a relatively steep learning curve. We recommend supervision, so that clinicians can maximize their learning and address concerns and issues that, in our experience, inevitably arise.

CHAPTER 9

Ending Treatment and Planning for the Future

Endings in therapy are often difficult, and that is especially true when the focus of treatment is on the complex traumas that attend combat. In all likelihood, adaptive disclosure has facilitated a meaningful engagement with traumatic feelings and memories and, in doing so, has given both therapist and patient a taste of how deeply and productively they can go together into profoundly upsetting material. Something that had seemed insurmountable has been engaged and, within that enormous effort, both people have made real contact with each other and with some of the poignant existential issues to which we are all vulnerable. Our experience is that substantive and meaningful work can be done within this short time frame, and that there is often more that can and should be done. Unless the focal trauma was fairly discrete and the patient's resources very high, at the beginning of the final session there will still be, in all likelihood, tremendous work to be done, and it is likely to be distressing to both patient and therapist to leave this work undone. In this chapter we primarily address how to optimize the ending, and we also touch briefly on how to profit from adaptive disclosure strategies when therapy is not limited to eight sessions.

As is the case with other trauma-focused psychotherapies, adaptive disclosure is designed to interrupt the automatic stream of toxic meanings and emotions triggered by traumatic memories and to replace dread, self-blame, hopelessness, and so forth, with a series of experiences that would drive the therapeutic work forward into day-to-day life, thereby facilitating a better adaptation over time. It is important that both the patient and the therapist remember that even if the therapy was powerful and positive, there will be challenges ahead. At the termination point, realistic expectations, followed by clarification and consolidation of the work that has been done, are critical to creating a mastery experience that can be the basis of further growth. The reviewing, clarifying and planning work of the final session is intended to highlight adaptive disclosure as a paradigmatic learning experience and to locate the individual work within a broader framework, elucidating ways in which new, consistently enacted behaviors, can plant the seeds of a more hopeful and productive future.

Concretely, the work of the final session centers on collaboratively reviewing and summarizing the process and progress of what has occurred. It is a time to get and to give feedback about strategies that were (and were not) productive and helpful, to review in-session and extrasession responses to the therapy, and to elucidate the broader implications of what has been learned, always underscoring avenues of more effective coping. Those behaviors that minimize the control of the present by the traumatic past, and create an increasingly robust base of life-affirming behaviors will be emphasized and there will be an effort to inoculate, as best as possible, against a resurgence of self-hate and despair, especially in the context of loss and moral injury. If there are referrals that need to be made, this is the time to do it. If the therapist has tracked PTSD (or other symptoms) weekly over the course of the therapy, these should be graphed and shown to the service member or veteran.

Throughout the last session, there should be an ongoing effort to locate the service member's individual struggle within the larger work, family, and social communities to which he or she belongs. The therapist should help link the patient's experience of the therapy and what he or she got out of it with his or her connection to the military culture and the veteran community, especially with respect to his or her professional role and identity. For example, when terminating, it will be important for therapists to help service members think about challenges that will arise in their military role (e.g., in their unit) and what they think they have learned that they can bring with them to that role and context.

The final session should cover the following topics and issues:

Reviewing and evaluating the work (giving and receiving feedback)

Appraising and normalizing incomplete healing and processing

Promoting adaptive functioning (e.g., self-care and reattachment)

Reviewing and evaluating the work (giving and receiving feedback)

It is will be helpful to begin the dialogue with a broad, open-
ended inquiry about the treatment, so that the service member or veteran is free to review his or her experience in any way that feels true.
This will provide the richest starting point, and there will be plenty
of opportunity to get more specific should issues not arise spontane-
ously. It may be necessary for the therapist to work actively to ensure
that the service member or veteran not feel pressured to be positive
in order to spare the therapist's feelings. This may require that the
therapist point out continued suffering or difficulty even if the patient
does not. The patient may be disappointed at what has not changed,
or surprised at how far they have come. In either case, it is important
to aim toward specificity and nuance—illuminating dynamic associations that the patient has made and helpful behaviors that have been
discovered, as well as noting continuing vulnerabilities that need to
be addressed.

A possible prompt for beginning the conversation might be as follows:

> "We are at the last session and you have met an extraordinarily dif-
> ficult challenge with tremendous courage. This is our opportunity
> to review the work that has been done so as to learn as much as we
> can from it and to use what we have learned to plan for the next
> stage. To begin with, what has this process been like for you?"

The emerging dialogue provides an opportunity to weave the therapist's observations together with those of the service member or veteran, and to deepen the work that has been done by defining and clarifying what has happened, and linking it to specific behaviors and ways
of thinking about the meaning and implication of the principal harm
processed in adaptive disclosure. Whereas Sessions 2–7 emphasized
intense emotional and "hot" cognitive processing, this session is the
time to anchor this work within the cooler, broader context of what is
known generally about life-threatening trauma, loss, and moral injury,

and recovery from these war-related harms. The therapist should not be afraid to teach a bit here and to link the patient's personal process to more general information where relevant. As the conversation proceeds, the therapist will want to focus on what has been learned, what has worked, and what needs to happen next.

The following are questions that might be used to stimulate the review:

"What have you learned? What did you get out of adaptive disclosure"?

"What has changed? What has not changed?"

"What will you take with you from our work together?"

"How do you feel about your ability to continue this process?"

"What do you think remains to be done?"

Appraisal and Normalization of Incomplete Healing and Processing

The therapist should inquire about things that remain difficult for the service member, as well as processes that were unhelpful in therapy, because both of these will guide the conversation about planning for future challenges and work that remains. If the patient hesitates here, the therapist can offer observations and interpretations that uncover these issues. Because of the severe, sustained, repeated, and grotesque nature of war trauma, loss, and moral injury, in many cases, there will be continued sources of distress, for example, in the form of specific PTSD symptoms, continued guilt, grief, shame, isolation, struggles with self-care, and compromised self-worth.

It is important for the therapist to be pragmatic and nonpathologizing. War is horrific, and it is absurd to think that residual suffering represents some kind of personal failing or that a brief psychotherapy can eradicate the painful legacy of combat. It is important to be respectful about the scope of the traumas that have been tackled and to frame the patient's suffering and courage within that context. If the therapy is coming to a close because of nontherapeutic forces (or before the patient wishes), that too should be honestly acknowledged. It is important to normalize and validate feelings of loss, anger, and anxiety (without getting unduly distracted by outrage, legitimate though it might be) and at the same time to be reassuring about the concern that the end of therapy means the end of progress. The patient's attention can be brought to the place that adaptive disclosure has created as an opening for a new experience or perspective. For example, once a service member or veteran understands that meaning is not inherent in a situation but rather is actively constructed through thought and behavior, a door has been opened to all sorts of new learning.

Furthermore, it will be useful for the therapist to shape the patient's conclusions, elucidating small (but significant gains) on the one hand, and highlighting continuing vulnerabilities on the other. For example, an appreciation of the reality that self-destruction is not a useful act of homage, or penance, is a step, even if it is not complete, just as a more complex and moderate appraisal of one's culpability is progress, even if it falls short of full self-acceptance. Any progress, no matter how small or partial, should be noted. The expectation is that what is learned will generalize, and typically, once something has been experienced, it is easier to do it again. It is important to emphasize that adaptive disclosure is not an end; it is the beginning of a means.

Therapists need to instill hope and applaud work accomplished, to be honest about what is left to do, and to be creative and persistent in constructing positive, valid, and emotionally plausible frameworks about what has occurred. It is important never to oversell what has been accomplished or to minimize residual pain. Merely sticking with the process and being willing to confront exceptionally painful emotions is a remarkable act of bravery and constitutes a success.

Most important is to assert that trauma gets healed primarily not through the dramatic anguish of an exposure or breakout component session but through the very persistent (albeit still difficult) practice of certain behaviors and ways of thinking to promote positive shifts in the meaning and implication of war-related harms. Throughout, the emphasis should be on an ongoing and continuing journey in which adaptive disclosure is merely one step.

Promoting Further Healing and Adaptive Functioning

The ways in which traumatic memories, thoughts, and feelings will continue to surface can be framed as a problem of past versus present. Referencing the ways in which memory and association works can destigmatize this phenomenon, as well as provide a useful model of how to modify it. In a way that is different from the exposure and experiential breakout components but entirely consistent with the processing and homework that has accompanied these components each step of the way, service members can be invited to think about what they can do to pair "opposite actions" with painful memories, such that, over time, the memory and its related thoughts and feelings are is modified. The goal is help the service member or veteran generate a plan of how to meet the inevitable activation of the past and the related impulses to act on those remembrances through, for example, self-hate (in all its manifestations), substance abuse, isolation, and avoidance. Patients can be encouraged to meet painful episodes with corrective self-talk that flows from what they have learned from processing and reframing the meaning and implication of their traumatic memories. They can also be encouraged to counter these experiences with other types of behaviors that pair traumatic activation with opposite actions, such as behaviors that engender calmness or positive absorption, so that, over time, their experience of the memory shifts.

There are many ways to proceed through this conversation, and all of it should be based on what the therapist and the service member or veteran have explored in the preceding weeks. For example:

> "Memories and painful feelings about military experiences will always be with you. And, they will continue to surface. Each time painful memories surface you have some choices about how to respond. You should know that your responses, over time, get attached to the memory and begin to change your experience of it. So, time is on your side, but only when you are actively and consistently engaged in changing your experience of the past. What are you going to take with you from the work we have done to help you respond to these challenges in a positive healing way over the long haul?"

It may also be useful to have a specific conversation about triggers. Certain triggers can and should be avoided (e.g., there is no particular reason to go to a war movie unless there is the desire to do so). Others should not be avoided (intimacy, children, self-care, etc.). It is important to make a distinction between temporary strategic avoidance (by choice) that stems from self-awareness, self-care, and acceptance, and avoidance that is automatic and uncontrollable, which confirms traumatic meanings and feelings (e.g., as pervasive isolation).

Additional prompts may include the following:

> "Let's take a moment and look at what you have learned about what triggers intense, unwanted, thoughts and feelings about [the principal harm]."

"Have you noticed any patterns in what causes you to think about [the principal harm] in ways that you do not want to?"

"How do you typically respond?"

"What can you do differently to help yourself moving forward?"

The focus of the ensuing conversation is on distinguishing healthy self-protective avoidance from maladaptive avoidance, as well as differentiating between mini-exposures, which are necessary and helpful, and situations that may be overwhelming and counterproductive, which are not. It may also be useful to distinguish baseline everyday coping with triggers (e.g., basic self-care, going for a walk or to a movie, or simply exposing oneself and finding ways to breathe through the activations that come one's way) from the red flags of seriously heightened symptoms (arousal or numbness that does not abate, dissociation, disordered eating, depression, substance abuse, rage, etc.) that may require larger actions, such as reaching out to specific people, or reengaging in various kinds of therapy. The end result of the conversation should be a list of potential triggers, resulting thoughts and feelings, and possible adaptive responses, as well as an understanding of what gets in the way of making these responses.

Promoting Self-Care

The therapist needs to educate the patient about the need for self-care, discuss specific means of taking care of oneself, and ask the patient for his or her own ideas on what he or she will do to stay healthy. A good night's sleep, regular balanced meals, moderate caffeine usage, exercise, and some regular practice that focuses and calms the mind should be emphasized. These behaviors are essential to well-being and, when done consistently over time, their impact is profound. They must be practiced assiduously when life feels relatively OK, then redoubled when life feels difficult. Since most service members and veterans know this, the necessary conversation here centers on impediments to self-care.

Some impediments are mundane and can be addressed simply by problem solving (sometimes one behavior that accomplishes the same aim needs to be swapped out for another). Also, explicating the importance of these behaviors for adequate functioning and, more importantly, itemizing their specific relevance to ongoing trauma work, can further heighten motivation. For example, one rudimentary prerequisite for trauma treatment is to live in a present that is different from the traumatic past, thereby enabling the past to be modified by a different context and a different set of associations (e.g., when an exposure experience in the context of life-threatening trauma is followed by reduced arousal and calm acceptance rather than catastrophe). The body is the context of our present lives, and what is happening in our bodies is part of how we bring meaning to everyday life. Reducing chronic overarousal and emotional dysregulation is pivotal to changing one's experience of feeling activated all the time and to thereby misinterpreting the present (and reexperiencing the past in the present) through the lens of the activation in one's body. Reducing physiological arousal also reduces one's susceptibility to being triggered, and this too creates room for new experiences in the present. Conversely, physical dysregulation in service members and veterans both recreates feelings of vulnerability, thereby heightening the likelihood of being triggered, and makes them prone to other medical and psychological illnesses of dysregulation. Clearly, if the patient is a service member redeploying, this may not be applicable, but anything that the service member can do to lower his or her floor of arousal reduces the risk of severe activation of trauma memories. Seemingly unrelated actions such as establishing some equilibrium though diet and sleep, regular exercise, and engaging in calming activities lower the floor. Basic mental hygiene, such as taking breaks when needed, having downtime, being thoughtful and self-protective in seeking out positive connections and avoiding destructive ones, and reducing unnecessary arousal (e.g., certain kinds of media) do the same thing.

However, for the most part, the impediments to self-care are psychological. For many trauma survivors, especially service members and veterans who are also victims of other kinds of interpersonal trauma (e.g., child abuse), the act of self-care, in and of itself, is a powerful traumatic trigger. Taking care of oneself can be experienced as an assault upon defenses (e.g., self-blame and self-condemnation) that are used to keep helplessness, grief, shame, and rage at bay. When the patient violates his or her long-standing equilibrium by taking care of him- or herself, he or she may well activate intensely negative thoughts and feelings (much in the way that becoming sober may trigger a flood of traumatic intrusions and feelings). This dynamic should be examined when relevant and various strategies are identified to arm the patient in his or her ongoing struggle toward self-care.

If loss is the principal harm, other prompts might include the following:

"Another reason for not taking care of yourself is that you may feel guilty for having a 'good life,' while your buddy is not here to enjoy such things. You may be reminded of the loss, and the feelings that go along with the reminders may feel too painful to address (e.g., 'My buddy loved playing basketball; it doesn't feel right to play basketball without him')."

"What do you think your friend would actually want you to do in this circumstance? What would you want if the situation were reversed?"

When the principal harm is moral injury stemming from perpetration, the following prompts may be helpful:

"Another reason for not taking care of yourself is that you may feel like you do not deserve a 'good life' after what happened, or that you deserve to be punished. But self-care doesn't mean rewarding yourself. Self-care is about behaviors that create the foundation for a productive life in which you have the capacity to make a contribution."

"If you were talking to (the moral authority figure), what would he or she say about you denying yourself some of the things that will help you to carry on?"

Here, it may be helpful for the therapist to validate the struggle that the service member or veteran is going through and to acknowledge (if true) that the jury may still be out as to whether he or she is ready at this point in time to embrace self-acceptance or commit to making some kind of positive contribution that synthesizes predeployment values and conceptualizations of self with what feels meaningful now. However, basic self-care need not be part of that decision. Failure to engage in basic self-care will come at a cost to others (e.g., spouses and children; fellow combatants, if the service member will be redeployed). In other words, doing these behaviors, mechanically, out of a sense of duty, even resentfully, will still be helpful. Patients can be engaged simply as a required life-sustaining activity that creates more independence, reduces the burden on others, and creates a foundation for more stable functioning.

Additional suggestions for service members and veterans who are unable to generate sufficient self-care ideas might include the following:

- Engage in basic sleep hygiene so as to facilitate getting enough sleep.
- Eat balanced (regular) meals; avoid excess sugar and caffeine.
- Exercise/walk outside/practice yoga.
- Pray/meditate/go to church.
- Attend community/base events.
- Play with children.
- E-mail a friend.
- Invite a friend or partner to do something.
- Listen to music/read.
- Watch a favorite movie or TV show.
- Get a pet.
- Find and engage in a hobby.

In all likelihood, therapists have fostered these kinds of wellness behaviors in homework assignments over the course of adaptive disclosure. The final session is simply the time to underscore, contextualize, and expand upon them. It is important to be candid about the fact that, while absolutely critical, self-care strategies will not eradicate in-the-moment suffering or erase posttraumatic symptoms. It is not a cure but rather a necessary base that makes good days possible, prevents bad days from turning into extended catastrophes, and minimizes destructive physical and psychological spirals.

Social Reattachment and Reengagement

Support from others is one of the most important factors associated with well-being. People who are comfortably connected to others tend to be healthier and happier, to recover from disease more easily, and to cope with adversity better than people who are isolated and lonely. Connecting, or reconnecting, to the social world may be one of the most important things a service member or veteran can do to improve his or her life. Positive, meaningful connections are associated with healing, and isolation is a prime component of downward spirals.

However, positive connections may also be very difficult. War trauma of any kind is malicious and interpersonal, and can poison any sense of easy connection to other people. Instead of comfort and joy, other people can activate intense feelings of aloneness, alienation, anxiety, rage, shame, and guilt, motivating avoidance and confirming one's initial sense of alienation, aloneness, and badness. Service members and veterans who have suffered traumatic loss may be afraid of connecting to someone for fear that they could suffer more loss, and both grieving patients and those suffering moral injury may feel guilty (or unworthy) forging new relationships. Coming close to another person also means coming close to oneself and this is fraught with difficulty when one's sense of self is contaminated with traumatic guilt and shame. Managing the storms of feelings and triggers within a relationship can also be difficult, requiring sensitive negotiation. Finally, while meaningful relationships are indeed reparative and nurturing, traumatized people may also find themselves drawn to and trapped in destructive relationships that exacerbate their sense of damage.

The final session is a time to revisit what has been learned about the patient's interpersonal functioning as illuminated by his or her symptoms, interactions with the therapist, postexposure and postbreakout component processing, and homework efforts. The work with the therapist should serve as partial reference point: Real-life relationships are not like therapy, but therapy is a relationship between two people and has some generalizability. The conversation should emphasize the importance of nurturing, meaningful connections going forward, identify avenues for further growth, and note the ways in which the service member's experiences might interfere. At the end of the conversation, the service member should have a sense of his or her needs, vulnerabilities, and behavioral strategies for navigating this territory.

Possible prompts might include the following:

> "What have you learned about the ways in which your experiences have affected your feelings and relationships with other people (from exposure/processing/homework efforts/relationship with therapist)?"

> "What small steps can you envision yourself making to nurture the relationships you already have/engage more fully with other people/protect yourself from destructive relationships and create room for positive ones?"

THE END OF THE ENDING: VALIDATION, QUESTIONS, AND REFERRALS

This is a time for the therapist to share something of his or her experience of the work and to acknowledge what has transpired, to express some gratitude for the honor of participating in this work, and to communicate respect and appreciation for what the service member or veteran has taken on.

It is also a time to invite any remaining questions and welcome contact in case questions should arise in the future. In the event that the service member or veteran expresses significant continued distress or inquires about continued services, provide information and a referral for accessing such services. Try to make referrals as much of a warm hand-off as possible, so that there is a sense of being cared for and of linking adaptive disclosure with subsequent work.

A NOTE ABOUT NOT ENDING AFTER EIGHT SESSIONS

If the therapist and the service member or veteran have some flexibility as to how many times they meet, this may indeed be fortunate. The task then becomes one of balancing the clinical utility of a strict time limit with the freedom to serve more fully the individual service member. Time limits have value because they force both patient and therapist to confront what any of us would reasonably want to avoid. We are wired to avoid horror, grief, despair, and unsolvable painful conflicts. From the patient's perspective, he or she has already met the trauma and failed at least once; otherwise, he or she would not be sitting in front of the therapist. From the therapist's perspective, no matter how well intentioned or intellectually convinced we are of the necessity of approaching traumatic material, the very things that make us useful to the other person, namely, our empathy, ensures that we will feel some of what patients feel, and this drives us, in ways both subtle and overt, away from facilitating this very intimate confrontation with the human and social tragedy of war. Thus, for both patient and therapist, structure, guidance, and deadlines are enormously useful ways of keeping the work close to the horror it needs to address. On the other hand, war trauma is enormously complex. Sometimes one simply cannot get to all the aspects of even one traumatic event. Often, multiple traumas are linked through systems of meaning and pain, and it is necessary to follow those threads if one wants to provide optimal therapy.

We do not know what adaptive disclosure would look like as a longer-term therapy. In general, our recommendation is to keep the overarching pattern of the eight sessions but to bring some flexibility as to how they are numbered. In other words, one might find that a particular principal harm is well-addressed in two to three processing sessions, and at that point, the patient is emboldened to take on something more complex. Conversely, someone might need many more sessions to process and work through one particularly difficult traumatic event. In both cases, we recommend punctuating coherent stretches of therapeutic work with a version of the taking stock, feedback, and framing work of the final session. Clearly, one would modify it so as to make it germane to the circumstance and not be unduly repetitive. Depending on the circumstances, in some cases, it might be no more than spending part of the session reviewing what has been helpful, then moving on to identify and conceptualize the next phase of the work. It may also be very useful to use this time to focus more extensively on what the service member is doing outside of sessions, with an emphasis on self-care and reengagement with others, and any relevant impediments to these behaviors. This is also a time when one can examine, if needed, some of the other issues that can emerge in a longer treatment. All of this will also inform subsequent processing sessions.

Regardless of when the feedback and evaluation session comes, the point is to take periodic pauses in order to evaluate critically what has transpired and what needs to happen for continued progress. This moment of taking a breath in the work allows themes and learning to be underscored, practices to be discarded or enhanced, working hypotheses to be appraised, and issues that do not fit narrowly within the guidelines to be addressed.

PUTTING CHANGE IN CONTEXT

Finally, after consultation with their therapists, whether patients choose to continue or stop the work, it is important for clinicians to emphasize the evolving and ongoing nature of recovery from trauma and to underscore how much of the work can only go on outside of therapy. Here, clinicians should show their humility and shared humanity. The clinician might say the following:

> "No person (regardless of his or her psychological status) ever really hits the mark. People may be more or less symptomatic, or more or less pleased with themselves, but the human enterprise of trying to live well is always a process of turning toward where we want to be. Criticizing oneself for missing the mark and focusing on what one did not do is almost always counterproductive (and different from a thoughtful analysis of a misstep). It directs attention to the wrong action and compounds a mistake with one

or another form of self-condemnation, leading to stasis. It's like stumbling while running. You can sit down and think about what a jerk you are, or you can roll that downward momentum into the next step, thereby continuing your run. The idea is to keep moving forward and when one veers off, the solution is to turn, in the next moment, toward whatever one has defined as the light, be it moving away from self-condemnation, engaging in more self-care, or reaching toward someone or some work that demarks a positive engagement with something outside of oneself. Thus, while the specific actions and behaviors that require ongoing practice are concrete, the guiding principal is to keep turning toward those actions that we know will be helpful and to do so with as much compassion, toward oneself and others as possible."

SUMMARY

In this chapter, we have provided didactic material that will help clinicians end therapy in the most helpful and hopeful way possible. As we said at the outset, we did not develop adaptive disclosure as a cure nor do we think a cure in the medical sense is possible for serious and sustained war zone harms. The goal is to start a process; in our opinion, the intent should never be to offer an expectation of the eradication of suffering and impairment as a result of any psychotherapy for war-related psychic wounds. Consequently, the final session is important because there needs to be a balance between reviewing what was learned and gains made, and a frank discussion of what is ahead over the long haul. The last meeting is often bittersweet for both patient and therapist. If we have provided a way forward, some hope that positive change is possible, that forgiveness and compassion are possible, then mission accomplished.

CHAPTER 10

Using Adaptive Disclosure When Prior Complex Trauma Is Present

Adaptive disclosure treats military trauma within a structured, short-term, and flexible model. We focus in this chapter on some of the issues that may arise when additional, serious, non-combat-related traumatic experiences enter the picture. In clinical practice, such experiences in a service member's past may be revealed during intake. Or they may arise when war zone harms are addressed with adaptive disclosure and other, often earlier, developmental trauma, is unearthed, affecting functioning and requiring therapeutic attention. It may also become relevant when non-combat-related trauma influences service members' or veteran's responses to military life-threatening dangers, traumatic losses, and morally injurious events and, as a result, the processing of these responses. Although adaptive disclosure was not developed or tested as a means of addressing nonmilitary traumatic experiences, these experiences do, on occasion, become highly relevant. This chapter addresses some of the possible issues and adaptations clinicians may want to consider when non-combat-related trauma becomes relevant *in the context of adaptive disclosure*. Because there are other evidence-based treatments to help people who present primarily with early complex trauma (e.g., McDonagh et al., 2005), our focus is on using adaptive disclosure after more recent index traumas have been adequately addressed. The decision to use adaptive disclosure strategies to target other traumatic injury should only be considered after consultation with the patient about treatment options and when there is a judgment that changing strategies would entail a disruptive shift in context.

The many kinds of non-combat-related trauma that service members and veterans may have experienced prior to and during their deployments may emerge during treatment for combat-related PTSD. However, we focus on just one for illustration, namely, childhood abuse or neglect. We have chosen this as our focus, because a history of maltreatment during childhood is not uncommon in military and veteran populations, childhood trauma is associated with affect regulation and relational problems that may significantly affect the course and outcome of adaptive disclosure therapy, and the clinical presentation of unhealed childhood trauma in an adult may be dissimilar from that of adult-onset traumas (e.g., those experienced during combat). It is our hope that by using this as our reference point, we can alert clinicians to issues and adjustments that may be helpful to consider for a variety of complex clinical presentations.

CHILDHOOD TRAUMA

The prevalence of premilitary exposure to potentially traumatic events is substantial, with estimates ranging from 35 to 57% (e.g., Rosen & Martin, 1996; Merrill et al., 1999). Many service members also have co-occurring non-combat-related traumas while in the military (e.g., traumatic loss, domestic violence, and sexual assault; Suris & Lind, 2008; Campbell et al., 2003). Of the service members who have experienced non-combat-related potentially traumatizing events, some will have endured experiences that are at the severe end of the continuum, such as family- and community-based trauma beginning in childhood and continuing over many years, involving highly toxic experiences such as chronic sexual and physical victimization (e.g., Cabrera, Hoge, Bliese, Castro, & Messer, 2007; Schultz, Bell, Naugle, & Polusny, 2006).

A child who is being seriously maltreated within his or her family grows up inside a toxic environment. Adapting to continual adversity is costly and can lead to a wide range of vulnerabilities and impairments that may (or may not) fall into clear categories or syndromes but which, nonetheless, are likely to present difficulty for the patient or become relevant in treatment (e.g., Briere & Scott, 2006; Edwards et al., 2005; Felitti et al., 1998; van der Kolk, Roth, Pelcovits, Sunday, &

Spinazzola, 2005). The consequences of adapting to chronic maltreatment and neglect may be reflected in, among other things, how an individual thinks and feels about him- or herself and others, the quality of interpersonal relationships, mood and affective disorders, and patterns of emotional and behavioral dysregulation (e.g., Herman, 1997; Briere & Spinazzola, 2005; Cook et al., 2005). Many of the children growing up in violent or neglectful circumstances demonstrate remarkable resiliency. They function at a high level, are successful in their military and civilian careers, and are able to engage positively in treatment. Nonetheless, others (including some who are successful) demonstrate enduring vulnerabilities: They may be vulnerable to mental disorders; bounce back poorly from stressors, demands, and military harms; and their early experiences may affect recovery and response to treatment (e.g., Cabrera et al., 2007). In addition, in a civilian context, many of the small percentage of patients who disproportionly frustrate clinicians, struggle in treatment, appear resistant, and have trouble forming a positive working relationship are people who have endured unimaginable cruelty during their most vulnerable periods of development (e.g., Linehan, 1993) and we assume this is likely to be true in the context of treating service members and veterans as well. We hope that bearing in mind the possible presence of serious nonmilitary trauma in the backgrounds of service members and veterans will enhance clinicians' empathy and compassion, motivating them to use extra care when treatment is more difficult and/or when the service member or veteran reexperiences thoughts and feelings associated with developmental trauma during the course of adaptive disclosure. In doing so, we hope to better prepare the reader to meet the needs of the service members and veterans who are likely to seek help.

APPLYING ADAPTIVE DISCLOSURE IN THE AFTERMATH OF CHILD ABUSE

Adaptive disclosure seeks to address the stasis induced by traumatic thoughts and feelings, and to facilitate the construction of a new narrative, new learning, and a pathway to healing over the long haul, especially in terms of hopefulness, self-care, self-compassion, and forgiveness. Like any short-term exposure-based therapy, adaptive disclosure is appropriate for people who can access conscious memories of their traumas, rather than re-experience them primarily through dissociative experiences and/or acting out.

When one considers applying adaptive disclosure to nonmilitary trauma, the basic tenets of the model remain the same: working by paradigm, taking into account the broad context from which meaning is derived, applying a structured yet flexible approach, using exposure to facilitate hot cognitive processing, employing imaginal experiential breakout exercises to provide emotionally salient corrective experiences, and consistently emphasizing self-care and positive connections with other people and activities outside of the sessions. What changes primarily are pacing and sequencing, cautions, and some of the nuances of the breakout experiential components.

Adaptive disclosure makes several demands on service members and veterans that may become progressively more difficult as the severity of the service member's or veterans' developmental trauma increases. Among these demands are tolerating intensely distressing emotions without losing authority over the memories that provoked them; simultaneously holding in awareness sharply contradictory beliefs, attitudes, and perspectives; and maintaining some capacity to empathize with themselves at different ages. When the focus of adaptive disclosure shifts to early life traumas, the clinician bears the responsibility to assess continually the capacity of the service member or veteran to meet the demands imposed by the treatment, shifting to other techniques as needed before there is a failure experience. A critical component of service members' or veterans' capacities to meet the demands made by adaptive disclosure is their alliance with the therapist and their ability to use the therapeutic relationship not only to endure distressing and disorganizing memories but also as a template for internalizing new self-regulation and self-care skills. Once again, the therapist bears full responsibility for monitoring the nature and quality of the therapeutic relationship in adaptive disclosure, including shifting to other approaches when breaches in that relationship require repair.

Other risks of using adaptive disclosure to treat developmental trauma deserve to be carefully and repeatedly considered. To the extent that early life trauma has negatively influenced the development of a service member or veteran, more weeks and months of therapy may be necessary to accomplish therapeutic goals. One risk is that the service member or veteran will be unable to complete the therapy, or get far enough along in it for the process to continue outside the clinical relationship. Often survivors of severe childhood abuse manage to compartmentalize what they have experienced. While this may be costly in certain ways, it may also engender successful functioning in other, critical ways. Opening up a childhood history of maltreatment, or another highly fraught and complex trauma, is potentially destabilizing, and this may be particularly risky within the context of military life. Life demands, such as those imposed by military training and operations, other employment, or the needs of family members, may place hard limits on the duration of therapy and the additional stressors and resources that are present during the therapy. The shorter the time available, the more modest the treatment goals should be. Especially for active service members, therapy can be interrupted at any time for any number of reasons, raising the risk that a service member will leave not only before the work has been completed but also perhaps when distressing and disorganizing memories and emotions have become intense and frequent, and this too must be taken into account in planning the work. Regardless of the duration of the therapy, when addressing early trauma, symptoms may get worse before they get better and functioning may therefore be temporarily compromised; this is likely to be particularly problematic within a military setting. This risk should be jointly borne by the therapist and the service member or veteran, taking into account everything that is going on their lives, now and in the foreseeable future. Sometimes, it may be prudent to delay therapeutic work on developmental trauma until the real-life consequences of a temporary worsening in functioning are lower. In such cases, the service member or veteran should be reassured that delaying is not the same as avoiding or quitting, drawing attention to the reality that even under the best of circumstances, the process of healing requires strategic planning and often a lifelong commitment.

In Chapter 4, we asserted that one of our working assumptions is that patients have within them the resources they need for the work of adaptive disclosure. While one's language in therapy can continue to be affirming, this may be an overly simplistic conceptualization of people who have grown to adulthood under the duress of chronic trauma, neglect, and betrayal, and more nuance and precision may be needed here. The risk of communicating to a service member or veteran the assumption that he or she possesses the internal and external resources needed to successfully complete the work of adaptive disclosure in the face of severe developmental trauma, when in fact, additional treatments and supports may be needed, is that thoughtful treatment planning may be diminished, adequate access to services and supports may be neglected, and there is a risk that the service member or veteran may leave the therapy ashamed and self-blaming or unnecessarily discouraged for failing to progress in treatment.

One of the potential core impacts of childhood abuse is the absence of internalized and positive attachment figures (i.e., empathic, compassionate, predictable) that may result in a diminished capacity for self-compassion, self-care, and the ability to form and maintain safe attachments (e.g., Herman, 1997). This may also engender distrust of authorities and others, reduced social support, and poor coping with life challenges, and it may also slow the development of the necessary therapeutic alliance. Childhood abuse can also restrict positive experiences and promote various kinds of tunnel vision, limiting one's capacity to hold alternative perspectives. These, as well as potential problems with emotional self-regulation, create an added risk of escalating nontherapeutic distress, acting out, dissociation, sharply increased symptoms, and problems with self-care and self-harm. As a result, survivors of child abuse often require a longer, present-day experience with a caring professional, a longer opportunity to develop a working relationship with a therapist, more in-depth skills development focused on self-care and emotional regulation, and more time to unpack the relevant aspects of their history and to develop skills at dealing with its emotional consequences (e.g., Cloitre, Koenen, Cohen, & Han, 2002).

Self-care may, in particular, present a conundrum. These seemingly positive behaviors may be potentially destabilizing and more elusive to enact in the aftermath of developmental trauma. More time may be needed to examine and respond to impediments to practicing these critical behaviors. Furthermore, in the absence of actual historical caring and protective figures, the therapist is more likely to have to play an active part in the imaginal dialogue, either by suggesting possible compassionate figures or by playing the role him- or herself.

Because adaptive disclosure is a directive approach that entails experiential strategies to promote self-compassion and self-forgiveness with service members and veterans, under some circumstances, for example, when the nonwar trauma is relatively limited or the patient's resources are very substantial, it may be appropriate to use adaptive disclosure as it has been described in this book to target a focal childhood harm. However, in the aftermath of severe and especially protracted developmental trauma, or in the presence of heightened vulnerability, we do not recommend eight sessions of adaptive disclosure as a stand-alone treatment. In these cases, consistent with the field at large, we recommend embedding adaptive disclosure within a longer-term treatment, so that the processing of traumatic material can be experienced within the context of a trusting and reparative relationship with a therapist. Also, consistent with other practitioners who advocate a sequential or phasic approach to treatment in order to create a base of affect regulation, safety, and self-care, we believe that the structured and active processing of traumatic material should, when possible, be preceded and/or supported by ongoing work to build these skills (e.g., Briere & Scott, 2006). Indeed, research has demonstrated the value of preceding the arduous work of processing complex trauma with a period of skills development focusing on affect regulation and interpersonal skills (see Cloitre et al., 2002; Linehan, 1993). This work is consistent with adaptive disclosure.

In general, when beginning to work with someone with a serious nonmilitary trauma, we suggest that one take extra time to gather and understand the patient's history (military and premilitary); get a sense of some of the primary themes of these experiences and the overlap between them; evaluate patterns of functioning, in particular, self-care, connection to others, and habits of coping; begin to define homework goals and anticipate (with the veteran or service member) potential obstacles; establish targets for adaptive disclosure; and educate and prepare the patient for the work. Each of these conversations provides an opportunity to validate and educate the patient, and to foster the connection between therapist and patient. Moreover, any in-depth conversation about childhood trauma is likely to be emotionally charged, providing mini-exposures and revealing important patterns of meaning and behavior that can be used to inform the subsequent therapy.

Sometimes survivors of child abuse respond to the invitation to address their history with the impulse to exhume the past as quickly and as completely as possible, so as to be done with it. Unfortunately, it does not work that way. The work of recovery is slow and incremental, and the exhausting, provocative work of processing abuse events and their meaning must be balanced with self-nourishment and positive connections with work and with people. It is as important to put the therapeutic work down, to turn away, and mindfully and compassionately to avoid unnecessary triggers as it is to approach the work in treatment and in other, carefully chosen ways. These two aspects of recovery must be balanced (Roth & Cohen, 1986). It may be helpful to emphasize explicitly that room must be made for positive engagements and to note that this requires some thoughtfully chosen efforts to turn away from trauma, in addition to the work of turning toward it.

Some suggestions that can be offered in this context include prompts such as the following:

"Recovery requires many different strategies, and all of them are important. For example, approaching these memories is necessary but it is also upsetting, difficult, and exhausting. It is real work, and like other kinds of work, it must be balanced out with adequate rest and with doing things that restore your strength so that you can keep doing the work, as well as live your life while you do it. This means that you must strive for a healthy balance of walking toward these memories and turning away from them. We have talked previously about the need to approach things that are very difficult. Let's talk now about what healthy avoidance and restorative activities are for you. What triggers do you want to avoid (and when and how) so that you can give yourself a restorative break? What other kinds of things can you do to replenish your reserves?"

Like other cognitive-behavioral approaches, an advantage is that adaptive disclosure facilitates approaching material that is difficult for both patient and therapist. Part of what makes the work tolerable is the structure and the implicit boundaries of the work. Yet one of the consequences of severe developmental trauma is that normal boundaries have been violated. This is true not only in the interpersonal world but also in the psychological one. Unbearable emotion, especially when it is chronic, tends to reside internally in an all-or-nothing state and especially when these feelings date from childhood, the threat of these feelings breaking through internal boundaries and spiraling into nontherapeutic distress can be real. Considerable attention should be paid to whether the patient has the capacity to process an event to completion and, in keeping with the paradigmatic approach of adaptive disclosure, to stick with the memory or issue the patient and therapist have decided to focus on (compared to moving from trauma to trauma in an escalating cycle of distress). Clear instructions may facilitate this for some people:

"It is important to take on these memories and feelings a little bit at a time. You may have the experience that focusing on one event leads you to think about another event, and so forth. This is normal, because the mind tends to link experiences that have something in common, so that things that feel the same are often associated with one another. Make note of these associated memories and please let me know what comes up for you, because it is very important to understand what things mean to you and knowing how thoughts, feelings, and memories are associated in your mind is part of how we find that out. However, once we have made note of these other memories, I may remind you that it is also important to process memories one at a time. If we take on too much at once, it becomes harder, so if a lot of memories begin to intrude, I am likely to remind you to direct your mind to the task of focusing only on the memory at hand."

While this effort at partition may or may not be under the patient's conscious control, clear intention and direction can be helpful. It may even be helpful to ask the service member to speak to these intrusive memories directly and to tell them that they will be attended to, just not now.

If someone is absolutely unable to maintain focus and one memory consistently leads to another and another in a spiral of increasing distress, then a short-term exposure-based strategy is not appropriate. Similarly, a significant dissociative response is a counterindication for the highly experiential, exposure-based adaptive disclosure strategies. In these circumstances, the patient needs much more time to develop basic skills and to more slowly explore his or her history in a less emotionally charged way.

Choosing a target memory is often a challenge when there are many adverse events, and this is especially true in the aftermath of chronic childhood abuse. Instead of focusing on the principal harm by inquiring about the worst and/or most currently distressing experience, we advocate beginning with a relatively less overwhelming childhood memory after creating a hierarchy of adverse experiences that are emblematic of the kinds of abuse endured (e.g., shaming, rejection, physical abuse, sexual abuse, neglect). The chosen memory should have significant emotional resonance but should not be among the most threatening memories available. Even relatively less traumatic memories are still likely to activate core, distorted schemas about self and world, as well as intense feelings of guilt, shame, and loss. By starting with a relatively less threatening memory, exposure and processing are less likely to lead to escalating spirals of distress and a loss of self-control, or dissociation, and the processing is more likely to be a success. This, in turn, facilitates learning that traumatic experiences can be partitioned and approached, and that new understandings can be derived in an incremental way. The resulting hope and feelings of mastery should enhance the person's ability to tolerate subsequent exposures.

The heightened risk of being overwhelmed and feeling out of control (i.e., nontherapeutic flooding) and losing contact with the safety of the present leads us to recommend that the therapist begin the raw processing exposure component by asking whether the patient would like to keep his or her eyes open. In child abuse, accessing intense emotions is often all too easy, whereas not becoming seriously overwhelmed can be elusive. Therefore, patients may need more contact with the therapist and with the present, even during the focus on the past.

In any complex trauma there is likely to be a melding of different issues. Often as one issue is approached and addressed, the next, more difficult issue surfaces. Most recollections of severe child abuse involve all three aspects of harm that adaptive disclosure addresses, and different aspects (e.g., loss and moral injury) of the same trauma may require processing. While this multifaceted quality is true of many traumatic experiences, it is particularly true when working in the aftermath of a complex trauma such as child abuse. The strength and the challenge of adaptive disclosure in the context of complex trauma is to concretize the broad swath of potential injury into a form that can be grappled with in a direct, visceral, and immediate way.

Therapeutic Foci

Life Threat

While some child abuse is, in fact, life threatening, even when the threat of actually dying is low, the fusion of utter helplessness and terror that children feel in the context of being harmed by abusive adults is so annihilating that it may feel life threatening and worse. In general, when the focus is on child abuse, the phenomenology of life threat is generally a gateway to other issues, such as the terror of being overwhelmed, and this terror often drives a pernicious form of self-blame and self-condemnation.

Unfortunately, in the aftermath of severe developmental trauma, there are many roads to self-blame and self-hate. Self-blame and self-hate can be a direct internalization of how the child was treated, but it can also be a defensive way for the child to protect him- or herself from threatening feelings of helplessness, grief, and rage. When adults abuse children, they obviate the implicit rules of a moral universe and sometimes, in an effort to restore the sense that there is some moral order, children blame themselves (e.g., Ferenczi, 1949). The fear of being overwhelmed by feelings of helplessness and fear can engender rigidly clinging to beliefs and behaviors that seem to hold those feelings at bay. The presumption of personal responsibility when there is no actual responsibility may also infuse later appraisals of culpability in combat, and it may undermine efforts at self-care.

The fear of being rendered helpless and emotionally overwhelmed that can be particularly acute for child survivors of abuse imbues the common fear of processing traumatic material with a particular and sometimes justifiable intensity. In the absence of the kind of internal resources and capabilities that come from adequate developmental experiences, and/or in the face of chronic horrifying abuse, the risk of becoming overwhelmed or unable to function is real and must be taken into account (through slower pacing, adjustments in the process, and enhanced support and skills development).

Loss

Loss often has a somewhat different focus in the aftermath of child abuse. It is usually not the focal presenting problem (although depression may be prominent), but it is likely to surface as a very important issue while dealing with other problems. Here, we are, for the most part, no longer talking about the actual death of a person but rather the painful loss of what might have been, that is, what a patient imagines could have been had he or she not been unjustly victimized. For people who are severely abused by other people in marriage or in childhood, the losses more often concern the loss of a possible alternative life: choices and experiences that might have been different had the person valued him- or herself, and lost opportunities and time that cannot be recaptured.

Similar to the consequences of combat, grief is often tied up with an enactment of relinquishing and punishing oneself. Being victimized by trusted caretakers is likely to taint one's sense of self and may, in the aftermath, may make one feel that it is impossible to care for oneself, to have one's own back, as it were. In the aftermath of severe abuse and/or in the process of therapy, there can also emerge an awareness of having behaved badly in ways that reflect this disconnection and disaffiliation with oneself. This disaffiliation with oneself is painful, in and of itself, it engenders poor life choices and self-destructive behaviors, and it may increase the likelihood of taking actions in adulthood that violate one's values, thereby leading to more loss, a sense of moral injury, and self-condemnation.

Loss also engenders resistance. People resist hope, self-care, and getting better because it puts them in touch with all that they have lost. One sees the landscape of self-destruction and lost opportunity much more clearly once one is no longer acting out. Taking care of oneself and seeking positive connections can be extraordinarily provocative and painful, because they require that one reclaim a self that may feel contaminated by having been victimized. This difficult process can be facilitated by acknowledging and grieving what has, in fact, been lost.

The challenge and strength of adaptive disclosure is finding a way to represent these losses so that they can be grieved directly and immediately, even when what has been lost is less concrete than an actual death. The process remains the same. The exposure can focus on an event (e.g., being raped, beaten, or psychologically abused). The postexposure processing should narrow in on the self-schemas and losses that have cascaded forward from that event. The postexposure breakout component can utilize an image of a younger self that the person thought he or she could protect and preserve but was forced to abandon; or there can be a dialogue with a part of self that focuses on memories of the service member or veteran acting against him- or herself or in violation of his or her values. If asked to have a dialogue with an earlier self, it may become clear how much the survivor blames that younger self for having been a victim, and the postexposure dialogue can provide a new, more adult perspective on this, facilitating an embrace rather than a rejection of the self. Photographs are particularly useful tools for facilitating this postexposure dialogue, as is writing a letter or talking to an empty chair. Again, the focus is on facilitating a grieving process that is as visceral and as immediate as the memories themselves, and that is linked directly to the goal of greater self-compassion and acceptance.

It may also be necessary to take on feelings of rage related to all the losses (and to the abuse in general). Outrage is appropriate and justifiable, and it can be productive, but only if it is processed and channeled so that it goes somewhere, rather than becoming a permanent feature of the emotional landscape. It can be useful to frame child abuse as a basic human rights violation and to think through what kinds of action could acknowledge this as the injustice it is and work toward ways to validate and redress it.

Moral Injury

Although the term "moral injury" is not typically associated with childhood abuse, the phenomenology is remarkably similar. When, as is typical in severe ongoing child abuse, the perpetrator(s) is a trusted attachment figure, there is almost always the sense, in the victim, that he or she has been complicit and is tainted with the evil of the perpetration itself, and is therefore morally deficient and bankrupt in terms of his or her goodness as a person. Even when the perpetrator is outside of the family, unless the child is rescued and cared for by trusted others, feelings of culpability, self-blame, shame, and guilt are typically part of the aftermath, as is the common and enduring confusion between feeling badly and being a bad person. Children and adolescents also do things that violate their moral standards (which, like those of service members, may or may not be reasonable standards). They may be angry and abusive to children or animals more vulnerable than them, and they often feel they have failed to protect or prevent harm to another—even when this was not possible; they may be forced to collude with their abuser while under his or her control and, as they get older, may act out in a variety of ways that they later do (and sometimes should) feel badly about.

These experiences, in and of themselves, are targets for treatment; they are also likely to be relevant to how these service members or veterans think and feel about their combat experiences. Service members or veterans who have been abused and have had experiences that led to a war-based moral injury may fuse these two experiences in a variety of ways. The irrational self-blame of childhood may distort and enlarge their beliefs about their responsibility in combat; acts committed, omitted, or imagined may well confirm their childhood belief that they are irreparably bad. Furthermore, severe child abuse often reduces people's capacity to respond adaptively to stress, which makes acting out in combat more likely and taking care of themselves afterward more difficult.

One difference between addressing moral injury in combat versus child abuse is the position of the therapist relative to the question of culpability. When focusing on childhood maltreatment and rape, unlike in combat, culpability is straightforward: The child can never be responsible for the abuse, just as a rape victim cannot be responsible for being raped. Beyond this, the tasks are similar to addressing moral injury in combat. The therapist facilitates a careful, reality-based parsing of responsibility (with a heavy emphasis on the age and situation of the individual at the time), and endeavors to move the patient toward the imperative of self-acceptance and compassion, and eventually to corrective action (which in the aftermath of child abuse is directed primarily toward care of the self but may also take on other social actions). Often, as one moves across the developmental trajectory, responsibility becomes more complicated, and here the work merges with the approach to moral injury that we use in combat.

Service members or veterans who struggle with moral injury and were also abused as children may have a particularly hard time seeing their responsibility accurately and taking care of themselves. As noted earlier, self-blame can function as a defense against overwhelming feelings and realizations. Overcoming the resistance to self-care can therefore bring in its wake intense feelings of helplessness, rage, or grief, and this can feel destabilizing and may be resisted for that reason. This dynamic benefits from a full airing, and the thoughts and feelings underlying the resistance need to be addressed in conversations about homework and postexposure dialogue and processing.

Here, again, having a dialogue in imagination with a *younger self* may be helpful, as may having the service member or veteran talk to some other imaginary child as if the child were him- or herself. Having the service member or veteran explain how their distorted beliefs came to be, and what they realize (as an adult) is actually true about their responsibility may help them incorporate a more reality-based understanding of their culpability.

One of the aspects of military culture that may render processing all of these issues more difficult is, of course, the tremendous emphasis in military culture on qualities that are directly at odds with being a helpless child, namely, power, self-control, personal responsibility, and autonomy. Childhood is a time of relative helplessness. This is a part of being human, and accepting this cannot be avoided. A related problem is that as acceptance of one's own vulnerability emerges, so too may an increased awareness of other peoples' vulnerabilities, including civilians in combat.

Homework: Self-Care and Engagement with Life

Previously, we referred to the need to reconnect to one's precombat self as part of the process of integrating the meanings of combat and moving forward. With child abuse, there is often no time when one was not being traumatized, so the issue is not reconnecting with a prior self, but rather obtaining more freedom from the constraints of the past in order to develop a more whole, self-caring, and competent self. Much of the work of overcoming the consequences of loss and moral injury in child abuse centers around the struggle with homework and in particular, self-care and positive connections to others.

For survivors of severe abuse, homework should be dedicated primarily to the tasks of self-care and creating (often new) positive engagements and connections. In all likelihood, far more time in session will be devoted to exploring the difficulties and resistance to this work. Educating patients about how one set of thoughts and behaviors can function to protect (albeit with harmful consequences) against what feel like more threatening feelings can be helpful here, as can asking them to explore what they might feel if, for just a moment, they did not hold themselves responsible for what has happened. For example:

> "Sometimes one set of beliefs or feelings function to protect us from a second set of thoughts and feelings that feel threatening, and this can occur in ways that get in your way and distort what is true. For example, what happens if you are wrong, if it wasn't actually your fault? Can you imagine this happening to another child? What would that be like? How would you judge it? Can you imagine what that child would think and feel? What would you say to them if you could?"

The principle here is the same as that in a conversation with a dead buddy that addresses directly the issue of honoring his or her death through self-negation, and in doing so, the individual fosters and experiences other perspectives.

SUMMARY

We have focused on childhood abuse to illustrate how adaptive disclosure can be modified to address other complex life traumas. The many threats to successful completion of adaptive disclosure that we have enumerated are more likely to appear in service members or veterans who have endured severe and complex trauma. With care and continual monitoring of the service member's or veteran's mental state, functional capacity, and constructive engagement in the therapeutic relationship, many of the core techniques of adaptive disclosure may be effectively utilized in the treatment of non-combat-related trauma.

Diversity of Military Missions, Organizations, and Relationships

In Chapter 3, we offered a rationale that adaptive disclosure therapists should strive for military cultural competency in order to maximize their effectiveness with service members, veterans, and their families. We also described the warrior ethos as a relatively enduring set of values and guiding ideals that are common to military cultures worldwide, past and present. Here, we expand on the ideas introduced in Chapter 3 by providing an overview of a few of the explicit elements of military culture, such as military roles, relationships, and organizational structures, that form the tangible embodiments of the intangible values and ideals encoded in the warrior ethos. Whereas the warrior ethos is common to all service members and veterans in all times and places, the explicit elements of military culture to be discussed in this appendix are highly diverse and unique to each of the thousands of roles service members perform in each of hundreds of military organizations that currently exist in the United States alone. Using a tree as an analogy, one may consider the trunk as a defining feature of the tree ethos; most trees have trunks, just as most warriors subscribe to the warrior ethos. But each species and variety of tree builds uniquely on the idea of a plant with a long, woody stem. Here, we take a 40,000-foot tour of the landscape of warriors and military organizations that exist today, each representing a unique solution to a particular set of military challenges, but all reflecting the warrior ethos as the tie that binds. This is not intended to be a comprehensive education in the diversity of military service. It can only provide a framework for each mental health provider to learn more about the unique experiences of every service member, veteran, and military family member in their care.

In the following sections, military diversity is described along these specific dimensions: missions, organizational structures, hierarchies, and social classes defined by rank. For more detailed information, see Module 2 of the VA/DoD online course, Military Culture: Core Competencies for Healthcare Professionals, available to the public at no charge (*www.deploymentpsych.org/military-culture*), and to VA employees on VA Learning University (*www.valu.va.gov/home/index*).

MISSIONS OF THE U.S. MILITARY

The official "mission" of the U.S. military is somewhat euphemistically defined by the DoD as the deterrence of war and the protection of the security of our country. Obviously, our military has not been used exclusively in passive deterrence and protection roles since it was established in 1775, and increasingly, the military forces of Western democracies have been deployed to perform missions that do not even involve combat—in the past sometimes referred to as "military operations other than war" (MOOTW) in the past—including growing numbers of humanitarian missions in countries beset by natural or man-made disasters. Figure A1.1 provides examples of military missions occupying the spectrum from peacetime to war.

A more comprehensive mission statement for the U.S. military could be written by imagining situations in the world in which core military competencies might be employed to good advantage in support of our national policies. Obviously, countering or deterring aggression would appear high on a list of such situations, but increasingly, military forces of

Peace	Conflict	War
• Humanitarian assistance • Disaster relief • Civil support • Nation building • Counter-drug support	• Countering terrorism • Support of insurgencies • Peacekeeping • Show of force • Containment	• Strikes, raids, and attacks • Limited warfare • Multinational warfare • Large-scale combat • Global warfare

FIGURE A1.1. Spectrum of military missions from peace to war.

the United States and its allies are deployed to trouble spots in the world not to destroy but to build and render aid. The Ebola outbreak in Africa is a recent example of a world problem that would be much harder to address without military involvement. The following are a few of the characteristics of the military that make it a useful instrument of American foreign policy—or of domestic policies, in the case of the National Guard—in so many different situations:

- Readiness: maintaining a high level of training, equipping, and partial prepositioning in order to respond as needed anywhere in the world, within hours or days.
- Mobility: having the ability to represent America anywhere in the world, on land, sea, air, space, or cyberspace.
- Modular flexibility: comprising organizational building blocks that can be assembled into a limitless variety of purpose-built forces.
- Logistics: having the capability to coordinate operations involving virtually unlimited numbers of people and quantities of supplies and equipment.
- Engineering: having the skills and tools to design and construct buildings, airfields, bridges, dikes, and just about any other needed structure.
- Autonomy: being able to conduct many operations with limited or no support from other entities.
- Security: being able to protect its own or other's people, equipment, and positions.

OVERVIEW OF MILITARY ORGANIZATIONAL STRUCTURES AND FUNCTIONS

The U.S. military comprises *three distinct organizational elements*, each with its own mission, structure, resources, funding, and chain of command: the DoD; the Unified Combatant Commands; and the four military Service branches (five, counting the Coast Guard). Understanding how they interrelate adds to military cultural competency in two ways: (1) It helps us better decode the accounts of military deployments and operations of service members and veterans, and (2) it helps us zero in on which organizational affiliations *matter* to the person telling his or her story, and which ones do not. As proposed in Chapter 3, love and honor drive much of the behavior of service members deployed to conflict areas, but both love and honor are intensely socially shared emotions. To understand the full impact of a any single military operational event, it is helpful to know up front for whom the person living through that event felt love and loyalty, and whose collective honor was at stake.

The relationship between these three strata of military organization is summarized in Figure A1.2; a more comprehensive organizational chart can be found at *www.defense.gov/orgchart/#v.*

Here's the long and short of it: Most military missions are executed by Joint Forces operating under the command of the U.S. Combatant Commander responsible for that part of the world (e.g., U.S. Central Command, responsible for the Middle East, the Horn of Africa, and Central Asia) or for that subtype of mission, if of limited scope (e.g., U.S. Special Operations Command, to which all Navy SEAL, Army Green Beret, and other special operators belong when deployed). DoD directs the Combatant Commander from the Pentagon, and the Joint Chiefs of Staff provide guidance, but it is the third organizational level where the rubber meets the road, and that matters to the individual soldier, sailor, airman, or Marine: that of small units, each containing between a few and a few hundred service members who trained together, operated as a team together during deployment, suffered hardships together, then returned home together as a unit. These are the indivisible atoms that comprise the substance of military forces. What small units are called (e.g., fire team, work center, or squadron), how they are constructed, and what they are trained to accomplish varies from community to community within each Service branch, but what they all have in common is the fact that they are all teams of persons who share a common identity and a bond of trust built on familiarity through shared hardships and successes. Service members do not love or cherish the honor of the DoD or the U.S. Unified Combatant Commands, and they certainly do not love or feel compelled to protect the reputation of multinational coalitions of which U.S. Joint Forces may form only a part. But they do love and cherish the honor of their companies and battalions on the ground, squadrons and flights in the air, and ships and boats on the sea.

The significance of the small unit for the mental health of the deployed service member is hard to overstate. Most of the risk and protective factors that influence mental health trajectories across deployments, and nearly all of the resources available for coping, reside within the small unit. Leadership and cohesion help the most at this level, and betrayals of trust and losses at this level do the most harm. One good way to learn about military small unit membership from a service member or veteran patient is to simply ask, "Who were you with?" or "What units did you belong to?"

THE FIVE MILITARY SERVICE BRANCHES

The Army, Navy, and Marine Corps were established by separate acts of the Continental Congress in rapid succession during the first year of the

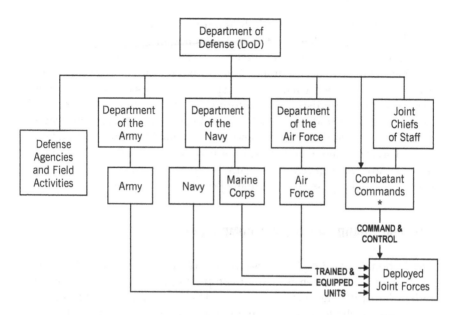

FIGURE A1.2. Warfighting organization of the Department of Defense (DoD): Service branches provide trained personnel and equipped units for Joint Force missions, but command of those forces is delegated by DoD to one or more of the nine Combatant Commanders: U.S. Combatant Commands: Africa Command (AFRICOM), Central Command (CENTCOM), European Command (EUCOM) , U.S. Northern Command (USNORTHCOM), U.S. Pacific Command (USPACOM), Southern Command (SOUTHCOM), Special Operations Command (SOCOM), Strategic Command (STRATCOM), and U.S. Transportation Command (USTRANSCOM).

Revolutionary War—the Army on June 14, the Navy on October 13, and the Marine Corps on November 10, 1775. These dates are celebrated every year as the birthdays of these three services. The cultural roots of the Army, Navy, and Marine Corps go back many thousands of years, dating to the first use of weapons by organized groups fighting on land or sea. The U.S. Air Force developed much more recently, of course, following the widespread use of aircraft in war. The Aeronautical Division of the Army Signal Corps, the first U.S. military aviation organization, was created on August 1, 1907, as part of the Army. The U.S. Air Force became a separate service branch on September 18, 1947, after World War II ended. The Coast Guard is the fifth military Service branch, because in wartime Coast Guard units may deploy for combat duties alongside units from the Navy, even though the Coast Guard belongs to the Department of Homeland Security rather than to the DoD. The Coast Guard is actually older than the Army or Navy.

On August 4, 1790, President Washington commissioned a fleet of 10 vessels to enforce tariff laws and to prevent smuggling, although the Coast Guard was not officially established by Congress until 1915.

Each military Service branch has its own encompassing culture and array of subcultures. Each uses its own particular set of tools and technologies; wears its own distinctive uniforms; speaks its own rich jargon; and exercises its own traditions, customs, and courtesies. There is no way to summarize all these differences, and no substitute for using every encounter with a service member or veteran as an opportunity to learn more about them. Figure A1.3 compares the Army, Navy, Marine Corps, Air Force, and Coast Guard along just a few of many possible dimensions.

NATIONAL GUARD AND RESERVE COMPONENT

The National Guard and the Reserves are often spoken of together, since they share the common feature of comprising part-time citizen-soldiers rather than full-time service members. That commonality defines many of the unique challenges of serving in the National Guard or the Reserve Component of one of the military Service branches. Whereas members of the Active component have no other job but to train, deploy, and redeploy (return home) with their small units, allowing for opportunities to develop and sustain great levels of trust and coherence as a team, members of the

Service Branch	Service Member	Highest Rank	Traditional Battlespace	Characteristic Platforms (Vehicles)
Army	Soldier	General	Land	Tanks, armored personnel carriers, helicopters
Navy	Sailor	Admiral	Sea	Ships, submarines, airplanes, helicopters
Marine Corps	Marine	General	Littoral areas (land near the sea)	Amphibious assault vehicles, tilt-rotor Osprey
Air Force	Airman	General	Air, space, cyberspace	Spacecraft, satellites, missiles, airplanes
Coast Guard	Coast Guardsman	Admiral	Domestic coasts and ports	Cutters, airplanes, helicopters

FIGURE A1.3. Comparison of the five U.S. military service branches.

National Guard or Reserve Component devote only a portion of their time to face-to-face contact with their military teammates before and after deployments. Hence, many fewer protective factors and resources may be available to a National Guard or Reserve Component member when he or she is not physically wearing the uniform.

National Guard and Reserve Components also differ in many important ways. Although the National Guard is overseen at the national level by the National Guard Bureau, jointly administered by the Army and the Air Force, the National Guard actually consists of 54 independently operating military organizations belonging to the 50 states and four territories. Unless mobilized and handed off to a Unified Combatant Commander for participation in a Joint operation, National Guard units operate at the discretion of their State governors. The Reserves, on the other hand, are components of the federal military Service branches, intended to be virtually indistinguishable from Active component personnel once recalled to active duty. National Guard units are characterized as either Army or Air National Guard; there are no Navy or Marine Corps National Guard units. On the other hand, all four branches of the DoD have Reserve Components. Title 10 of the United States Code (USC) regulates the organization and functioning of both Active and Reserve components of the military Services, as well as that of the federal National Guard Bureau. On the other hand, Title 32, USC, regulates the National Guard across the states and territories.

MILITARY HIERARCHIES

Military organizations are explicitly hierarchical. At every given moment, almost everyone in the military knows to whom he or she is subordinate, and who is subordinate to him or her—to whom he or she is accountable, and for whom he or she is responsible. Hierarchies reduce the friction that would otherwise be generated by persons competing for dominance and control at every twist and turn; in the military, it is clear who is in charge in nearly every situation. Hierarchies facilitate high levels of teamwork by unambiguously defining individuals' roles and the relationships between them. Many civilian organizations, from businesses to religions, are also hierarchical in structure, but military hierarchies have a few distinctive features.

Military Rank versus Position

Military groups are organized along two simultaneous hierarchical dimensions: by "rank" (defined at the level of the institution) and by "position" (defined at the level of the small unit). Every military rank has its place in the rank continuum, from recruit to general or admiral, and relative ranks are important for the proper exercise of military customs and courtesies—for example, in determining whether two service members who pass each on a sidewalk should salute, and if so, who should salute first. Rank also partly determines pay grade, benefits, and other important aspects of military life. But rank hierarchies rarely, if ever, determine who is in charge, who has authority over the other members of the group, and who is responsible for not only for getting the job done but also preserving the health and well-being of unit members along the way. Authority and responsibility are defined not by rank but by assigned position in the unit. Every military unit of any size has an assigned leader and assigned second in command, and everyone knows and respects it. Most assigned leaders hold a higher rank than their subordinates, but not always. Positional seniority always trumps rank, even though a leader may address a higher-ranking subordinate as "Sir."

Military Rank and Position Matter 24/7

Hierarchies in civilian organizations tend to have a limited scope: They tend to operate only at certain times, such as during specific ceremonies or formal meetings. Military hierarchies, on the other hand, operate every minute of every day, whether on- or off-duty, and they often endure in the hearts of veterans long beyond their active military service. In each assignment in the military, service members know who they are fighting for, who has their back, who they wish to emulate. The CO (commanding officer) of a ground combat unit, such as an infantry battalion, will remain the CO of that battalion in perpetuity in the minds and hearts of the members of that unit.

Military Hierarchies are Transparent

One of the distinguishing features of military hierarchies, when compared to civilian hierarchies, is their transparency: A quick glance at a fellow service member's military uniform reveals one's hierarchical position relative to him or her, at least in terms of rank, institutional seniority, and experience—all easily read from the collar devices, ribbons, and other military bling, especially on dress uniforms. Civilian hierarchies are not as easily discerned and are confined to more limited aspects of group members' lives, such as only in the workplace, church, school, club, or family.

Military Leaders Make Life and Death Decisions

Another fundamental distinction between military and civilian hierarchies is the extent to which authority over life and death is invested in leaders.

In the military, especially in wartime, subordinates may be ordered to kill or maim other humans or animals, or to forfeit their own lives and limbs, at any moment, by superiors whose authority all service members have solemnly sworn to respect in their oaths of enlistment or commissioning. Many professionals in other walks of life bear life-and-death responsibilities; firefighters, police, and health care professionals are examples. But in few, if any, other professions do leaders make decisions that may cost the lives of healthy young men and women, in the prime of their lives, who are well-known and even beloved by the leader making those decisions. In few other professions are such decisions made by one person, acting alone and under extreme pressure, with few other persons to help shoulder the blame afterward. Nowhere else are the people making such life-and-death decisions mere children or just barely adults. Fortunately, military Services all have time-tested and proven methods for developing leadership skills in their members, so that the vast majority of decisions made in a war zone are probably sound, both tactically and morally.

MILITARY SOCIAL CLASSES

Military organizations have distinct social classes based on rank, but these are not social castes; after all, the military is a prototypical meritocracy that encourages great upward mobility, including the freedom to transition from one military rank group to another based on education, experience, and performance. As diagrammed in Figure A1.4, the two major social classes in the military are *officer* and *enlisted*. Officers are persons in whom a military institution has invested the highest levels of authority and responsibility, or who possess technical knowledge and skills that require many years of education and training. Officers usually have at least one undergraduate degree, and many have completed postgraduate education and training. Enlisted service members do not, in general, possess as much authority or responsibility, except as is delegated to them by the officers appointed over them. The officer-enlisted distinction is of fundamental importance in the military for defining what types of social interactions are permissible and which are not among service members. *Fraternization* is a serious offense for officers in the military, defined in Article 134 of the Uniformed Code of Military Justice (UCMJ) as a relationship of apparent equality between an officer and an enlisted person that could jeopardize good order and discipline in the military organization. Examples of fraternization including romantic or business involvements of any kind, or even friendships that blur the officer-enlisted boundary.

The stark divide between the officer and enlisted ranks in the military may seem like it is founded on the view that people of certain classes are

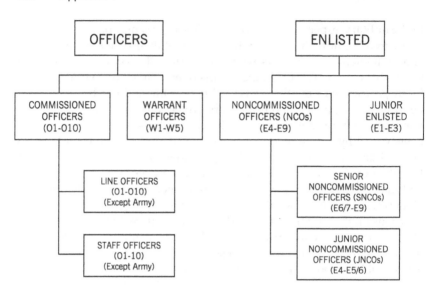

FIGURE A1.4. U.S. Military rank groups.

inherently worth more or less than those of other classes, such as is found in social caste systems. A better analogy to help make sense out of military rank classes is the distinction between parent and child in a healthy family. Good parents who love their children do not think for a moment that they are somehow better or more valuable than their own sons and daughters, but they also know their children's emotional and moral development depends on a firm yet flexible apportionment of authority in the family.

Drilling down further, both officer and enlisted rank classes include distinct subclasses, each with its own defining features. There are two broad subtypes of officers in the U.S. Military: commissioned officers and warrant officers. Commissioned officers comprise the vast majority of all nonenlisted personnel in the military; they occupy the full spectrum of roles in military units, up to and including command. In contrast, warrant officers are a small subgroup, comprising less than 10% of the U.S. military; their members tend to serve in technical roles, either as advisors to commanding officers or as practitioners of a technical craft, as in the case of warrant officer pilots in the Army. In the Navy, Marine Corps, Air Force, and Coast Guard, there are two major subgroups of commissioned officers defined entirely by their eligibility to assume command of operational military units, such as battalions, squadrons, and ships. Officers who are eligible for warfighting command have historically been termed "line officers," perhaps dating back to the times of wooden ships (also called ships of the line), which tended to fight battles in a long fore-and-aft line. Commissioned officers in these Service branches who are not eligible for accession to command of a warfighting unit are called "staff" officers; they include practitioners of any of a number of occupational specialties that are less directly military in their nature, including lawyers, physicians, dentists, and supply and repair specialists. Line officers are trained, from their first day of service, to command troops in battle; staff officers are not. The U.S. Army does not draw this distinction between line and staff officers based on eligibility for warfighting command.

Enlisted service members include two broad subgroups: junior enlisted (comprising the first three enlisted ranks), and noncommissioned officers (NCOs; typically beginning with the fourth enlisted rank), termed a Corporal, Specialist, Petty Officer Third Class, or Senior Airman, depending on Service branch. Of all class distinctions in the military, this one may have the greatest consequence for the lives of service members. Junior enlisted in the first three ranks have relatively little responsibility for other people; they are generally followers, not leaders. But once one advances to the fourth enlisted rank, everything changes. Corporals in the Army or Marine Corps are the men and women who lead the small teams that actually perform operational military missions on the ground, making decisions on the fly, often without the opportunity to seek advice or direction before taking action. The huge importance of NCOs to the success or failure of military missions, especially in counterinsurgency warfare, was captured by former Marine Corps Commandant, General Charles C. Krulak, in an essay he wrote in 1999 entitled, "The Strategic Corporal: Leadership in the Three Block War," available for download from *www.au.af.mil/au/awc/awcgate/usmc/strategic_corporal.htm.* "Three Block War" is a euphemism for the amorphous and complex conflicts of the current era; the idea is that on three contiguous city blocks in a third-world city, U.S. and allied troops may simultaneously be charged with executing three very different military missions: humanitarian assistance, peacekeeping, and traditional warfighting. Such complex military efforts may ultimately prove impossible. Think "Blackhawk Down" in Mogadishu or the UN response to the Rwanda genocide. Now realize that the most important decisions are often made in such operations by corporals and sergeants who are the same age as college kids partying on spring break.

Most Service branches divide the large group of NCOs, the backbone of the military, into junior NCOs (E4 to E5 or E6, depending on Service branch), and senior (or staff) NCOs (SNCOs; E6 or E7 and above). In all Service branches, SNCOs bear much greater responsibility than junior NCOs; they manage and lead more people and are responsible for larger military subunits. The most senior (E9) SNCOs, called Sergeants Major in the Army and Marine Corps, Master Chief Petty Officer in the Navy and

Coast Guard, and Chief Master Sergeant in the Air Force, function as advisors to the most senior commanding officers, representing the interests of all enlisted persons in their units. But the difference between SNCOs and more junior NCOs is not nearly as great as the difference in the weight of responsibility between a Corporal (E4) and a Private First Class (E3) in the Army, or between a Third-Class Petty Officer (also E4) and a Seaman (also E3) in the Navy.

Military rank groups are arguably true social classes in that they confer relative status. Uniforms, pay scales, assigned housing, traditions, and courtesies such as saluting all recognize the service member's position in one of these rank groups. But they are not social castes. Movement between social classes is both encouraged and expected, and no one in the military is considered more or less valuable than anyone else. Ideally, everyone has everyone else's back. The Marine Corps has a tradition that illustrates the strong vertical ties that bind Marines across ranks: on November 10, every year at every Marine Corps base around the world, the birthday of the Marine Corps is celebrated by the cutting of a birthday cake with a ceremonial sabre held by two Marines, always the youngest and oldest present.

The Meaning and Implication of Key Events Form

Please take a few moments to get into the right frame of mind to do this exercise. Find a private quite place and take some deep slow breaths. Try to free yourself from the day's demands and pressures. Give yourself at least 30 undisturbed minutes for this task.

Once you are in the right place, take just a few minutes and focus your thoughts on the military experience that has affected you the most; the event that is most currently distressing and haunting. Do not focus on details, but on the fact that this thing happened. After doing this, use this form to write about *what this experience means to you* and *what is the implication of this experience* in terms of: (1) your *beliefs about yourself* (e.g., your self worth, identity as a service member, or veteran, family member or friend, and so on); (2) *your beliefs about others* close to you (e.g., their trustworthiness); and (3) *your beliefs about how things work in the world* (e.g., fairness, justice). Feel free to write about any other issues that come to mind about the meaning and implication of this event. You do not need to fill all of these pages. Please bring this sheet with you to the next session.

Calming and Attention Focusing Techniques

In this appendix, we provide instructions for deep breathing and grounding strategies that clinicians can use to help patients manage in- and extrasession intense distress and loss of control, when applicable. The deep breathing content can be fashioned directly into a handout. The grounding instructions are written for clinicians to address in-session loss of control and severe dissociation.

DEEP, SLOW, DIAPHRAGMATIC BREATHING

When we are tense or anxious, our muscles tense up and our breathing becomes *faster* and *shallower*. This response is hardwired; our bodies are getting ready to respond to a challenge or threat (this is called the "flight-or-fight response"). Fast breathing helps us survive serious threats by rapidly supplying oxygen to our muscles. However, if there is no real challenge or threat (i.e., if one's life is not immediately in danger), one can "overbreathe," which can bring on a number of physical sensations that include feeling out of breath and lightheaded or dizzy, and having a rapid heartbeat or chest pains. An effective way to reduce tension and help calm the mind is to practice deep, slow "diaphragmatic" breathing.

Benefits of learning this type of breathing

1. It is very easy to learn and one can use this skill anytime, anywhere.
2. It helps one relax and manage tension and anxiety.
3. It helps one manage the times when one is triggered to recall distressing war experiences.

Learning relaxation skills does not hurt one's ability to respond to serious and real threats when one needs to do so. This skill will only enhance one's ability to take care of oneself in any situation, in part because it helps one to be rested and ready for the next challenge.

The goal is to use the diaphragm (a large muscle underneath the lungs, near the base of the ribs), to breathe while inhaling and exhaling *deeply and slowly*. When one breathes in using the diaphragm, one's stomach extends all the way out as the abdomen expands. Upon exhaling, one's abdomen is sucked back in as the stomach returns to its resting state.

Using the diaphragm for deep slow breathing is different than breathing from the top of one's chest. When one is tense or anxious, one uses the small muscles between the ribs and those at the top of the chest to fill the lungs. This changes the balance of oxygen and carbon dioxide in the body by bringing in too much oxygen and depleting too much carbon dioxide. Deep, slow diaphragmatic breathing counters this process. Breathing slowly and deeply from the diaphragm also slows down the heart rate, helping one to reduce tension and anxiety.

Deep breathing is a skill that needs to be practiced. The practice of periodic deep breathing generally lowers stress. Once a person is good at it, another important benefit is applying deep breathing when one needs it most, during states of very high emotion or distress, when one feels things going out of control.

How to practice deep breathing

- Find a quiet, comfortable place where you won't be disturbed.
- *Slowly* breathe in cool, calming air, pushing your stomach out near your belly button. Keep your chest still.
- Exhale slowly and deliberately. Pause naturally between each breath.
- Breathe slowly but naturally, keeping each breath smooth and easy.

Many people find it easiest to breathe through their nose, but do whatever feels most comfortable and natural for you.

- When you breathe in, think the word "one" to yourself. Then, breathe out slowly and think the word "relax." On your next breath, think "two" as you breathe in, and "relax" as you breathe out. Continue counting until you reach "ten," then start over until you get to "ten" again.
- Do this exercise for a total of *at least 1 minute.*

When you practice, as yourself: How do you feel now? Compare how you feel now to the tension you felt when you began. Do you feel more clearheaded and relaxed? Do you have any more energy than you had when you began the activity?

Tips for deep breathing

- Place one hand on your chest and one hand over your belly button. Breathe in and out so that only the hand on your abdomen moves, while the hand on your chest stays still.
- If you are having trouble breathing from your diaphragm, try "leading" each breath by pushing your stomach out. By making space for the air to fill, you are creating a natural vacuum that will draw the air in.
- If you are still having trouble, try practicing while lying on your back on the floor. Put a book on your belly and practice moving it up and down with each breath.
- It is important that you practice regularly, meaning *at least* once a day. The more you do it, the easier it will become, and the more you will benefit.
- You may not notice much difference in how relaxed you feel after you have done the breathing exercises today, but the more you practice, the calmer you'll feel in situations that do not require you to be "geared up" and tense.
- As you get comfortable with slow deep breathing, try practicing it for *longer* periods of time and in *different situations.* For example, try it while you are sitting in traffic, standing in the checkout line, watching TV, or walking (you can time your breaths to your steps). The more you practice in different situations, *the better you will be at relaxing yourself whenever and wherever you need to do so.*

If at first you find the exercise difficult or frustrating, do not give up—deep breathing gets easier with time and practice. Your body may have been operating on "high alert" status for a while now, so you need to be patient as you train your body to relax and "reset" itself to a more relaxed level.

Once you have practiced this exercise several times (e.g., daily for at least a week or two), you can start to use this skill to manage times when you are triggered to recall distressing or painful combat and operational experiences, or when you are feeling anxious or angry. As soon as you notice that you are upset, try to step back from the situation and focus on taking slow deep breaths for as long as you need to, in order to calm down.

Taking control of breathing is a good way to calm down and restore focus. This is one reason that breathing is stressed in martial arts; it creates a body–mind connection. This connection helps control how well the body receives oxygen, reduces stress, and increases self-awareness. Controlled breathing allows people to gain control over their bodies, including emotional reactions.

GROUNDING

In exposure therapy and adaptive disclosure, strong feelings are important change agents. Feelings need to run their natural course before they will subside, and there are times when it is safe and appropriate to do this. At other times, service members or veterans may need to maintain control over their emotions and focus on the task at hand. When a service member or veteran is so intensely immersed in an emotional experience that it is detrimental, the following *grounding* strategies can be used to restore focus. Therapists can guide patients through these steps to help them regain a sense of place and time, and to create distance, if necessary. Service members and veterans should also learn these strategies so that they can apply them when necessary in their lives outside the therapy context.

Keep your eyes open as you prepare to turn your attention from your inner world of distress to the calmer outside world. Look around you and see that you are safe—that there are no immediate threats to your life or safety. Notice that the thoughts and feelings that have made you feel unsafe do not belong where you are now. Now try to imagine putting a barrier between you and all of your unsafe feelings by wadding them up, stuffing them into a container, and sealing it. Next, imagine the container of your unsafe feelings being placed behind a thick concrete barricade far away from you.

Now look around the place where you are and name as many objects and colors as you can, one by one. Notice and name what is in front of you, to your left, to your right, behind you, above you, and beneath you. If you see any printed words, read them, then name each letter backward. Now focus your thoughts on naming things you are interested in (e.g., sports teams, types of dogs, the names of entertainers or athletes, or TV shows). Count slowly forward (1 to 10) or backwards (10 to 1). Notice the pressure of your body on the ground or floor. Stretch and take a deep breath.

Check in with yourself, and if you are still feeling unsafe or your thoughts are unclear and unfocused, repeat these exercises.

References

American Psychiatric Association. (2013). *Diagnostic and statistical manual of mental disorders* (5th ed.). Arlington, VA: Author.

Barnes, J. B., Dickstein, B. D., Maguen, S., Neria, Y., & Litz, B. T. (2012). The distinctiveness of prolonged grief and posttraumatic stress disorder in adults bereaved by the attacks of September 11th. *Journal of Affective Disorders, 136*(3), 366–369.

Becker, C. B., Zayfert, C., & Anderson, E. (2004). A survey of psychologists' attitudes towards and utilization of exposure therapy for PTSD. *Behaviour Research and Therapy, 42*(3), 277–292.

Boelen, P. A., & Prigerson, H. G. (2007). The influence of symptoms of prolonged grief disorder, depression, and anxiety on quality of life among bereaved adults. *European Archives of Psychiatry and Clinical Neuroscience, 257*(8), 444–452.

Boelen, P. A., & van den Bout, J. (2005). Complicated grief, depression, and anxiety as distinct postloss syndromes: A confirmatory factor analysis study. *American Journal of Psychiatry, 162*(11), 2175–2177.

Boelen, P. A., Van Den Hout, M. A., & Van Den Bout, J. (2006). A cognitive-behavioral conceptualization of complicated grief. *Clinical Psychology: Science and Practice, 13*(2), 109–128.

Bonanno, G. A., Moskowitz, J. T., Papa, A., & Folkman, S. (2005). Resilience to loss in bereaved spouses, bereaved parents, and bereaved gay men. *Journal of Personality and Social Psychology, 88*(5), 827–843.

Bonanno, G. A., Wortman, C. B., Lehman, D. R., Tweed, R. G., Haring, M., Sonnega, J., et al. (2002). Resilience to loss and chronic grief: A prospective study from preloss to 18-months postloss. *Journal of Personality and Social Psychology, 83*(5), 1150–1164.

Bradley, R., Greene, J., Russ, E., Dutra, L., & Westen, D. (2005). A multidimensional meta-analysis of psychotherapy for PTSD. *American Journal of Psychiatry, 162*(2), 214–227.

Briere, J. N., & Scott, C. (2006). *Principles of trauma therapy: A guide to symptoms, evaluation and treatment.* Thousand Oaks, CA: Sage.

Briere, J. N., & Spinazzola, J. (2005). Phenomenology and psychological assessment of complex posttraumatic states. *Journal of Traumatic Stress, 18*(5), 401–412.

Cabrera, O. A., Hoge, C. W., Bliese, P. D., Castro, C. A., & Messer, S. C. (2007). Childhood adversity and combat as predictors of depression and posttraumatic stress in deployed troops. *American Journal of Preventive Medicine, 33*(2), 77–82.

Cahill, S. P., Rothbaum, B. O., Resick, P. A., & Follette, V. M. (2009). Cognitive-behavioral therapy for adults. In E. Foa, T. Keane, M. Friedman, & J. Cohen (Eds.), *Effective treatments for PTSD: Practice guidelines from the International Society for Traumatic Stress Studies* (2nd ed., pp. 139–222). New York: Guilford Press.

Campbell, J. C., Garza, M. A., Gielen, A. C., O'Campo, P., Kub, J., Dienemann, J., et al. (2003). Intimate partner violence and abuse among active duty women. *Violence Against Women, 9*(9), 1072–1092.

Chen, J. H., Bierhals, A. J., Prigerson, H. G., Kasl, S. V., Mazure, C. M., & Jacobs, S. (1999). Gender differences in the effects of bereavement-related psychological distress in health outcomes. *Psychological Medicine, 29*(2), 367–380.

Cigrang, J., Peterson, A., & Schobitz, R. (2005). Three American troops in Iraq: Evaluation of brief exposure therapy treatment for the secondary prevention of combat-related PTSD. *Pragmatic Case Studies in Psychotherapy, 1,* 1–25.

Cloitre, M., Koenen, K. C., Cohen, L. R., & Han, H. (2002). Skills training in affective and interpersonal regulation followed by exposure: A phase-based treatment for PTSD related to childhood abuse. *Journal of Consulting and Clinical Psychology, 70*(5), 1067–1074.

Coker, C. (2007). *The warrior ethos: Military culture and the war on terror.* New York: Routledge.

Cook, A., Spinazzola, J., Ford, J., Lanktree, C., Blaustein, M., Cloitre, M., et al. (2005). Complex trauma in children and adolescents. *Psychiatric Annals, 35,* 390–398.

Cuijpers, P., Van Straten, A., & Warmerdam, L. (2007). Behavioral activation treatments of depression: A meta-analysis. *Clinical Psychology Review, 27*(3), 318–326.

Department of Veterans Affairs (VA). (2009). Understanding military culture. Retrieved from *www.ptsd.va.gov/professional/continuing_ed/military_culture.asp.*

Dohrenwend, B. P., Turner, J. B., Turse, N. A., Adams, B. G., Koenen, K. C., & Marshall, R. (2006). The psychological risks of Vietnam for U.S. veterans: A revisit with new data and methods. *Science, 313,* 979–982.

Dollard, J., & Miller, N. E. (1950). *Personality and psychotherapy: An analysis in terms of learning, thinking, and culture.* New York: McGraw-Hill.

Edwards, K. (1990). The interplay of affect and cognition in attitude formation and change. *Journal of Personality and Social Psychology, 59,* 202–216.

Edwards, V. J., Anda, R. F., Dube, S. R., Dong, M., Chapman, D. F., & Felitti, V. J. (2005). The wide-ranging health consequences of adverse childhood experiences. In K. Kendall-Tackett & S. Giacomoni (Eds.), *Child victimization: Maltreatment, bullying, and dating violence prevention and intervention* (pp. 8-1–8-12). Kingston, NJ: Civic Research Institute.

Ehlers, A., & Clark, D. M. (2000). A cognitive model of posttraumatic stress disorder. *Behaviour Research and Therapy, 38*(4), 319–345.

Felitti, V. J., Anda, R. F., Nordenberg, D., Williamson, D. F., Spitz, A. M., Edwards, V., et al. (1998). Relationship of childhood abuse and household dysfunction to many of the leading causes of death in adults: The Adverse Childhood Experiences (ACE) study. *American Journal of Preventive Medicine, 14,* 245–258.

Ferenczi, S. (1949). Confusion of the tongues between the adults and the child. *International Journal of Psychoanalysis, 30,* 225–230.

Foa, E. B., Ehlers, A., Clark, D. M., Tolin, D. F., & Orsillo, S. M. (1999). The posttraumatic cognitions inventory (PTCI): Development and validation. *Psychological Assessment, 11,* 303–314.

Foa, E. B., Hembree, E., & Rothbaum, B. O. (2007). *Prolonged exposure therapy for PTSD: Emotional processing of traumatic experiences therapist guide.* New York: Oxford University Press.

Foa, E. B., Keane, T., Friedman, M., & Cohen, J. (2008). *Effective treatments for PTSD: Practice guidelines from the International Society for Traumatic Stress Studies.* New York: Guilford Press.

Foa, E. B., & Kozak, M. J. (1986). Emotional processing of fear: Exposure to corrective information. *Psychological Bulletin, 99*(1), 20–35.

Foa, E. B., & Meadows, E. A. (1997). Psychosocial treatments for posttraumatic stress disorder: A critical review. *Annual Review of Psychology, 48,* 449–480.

Foa, E. B., & Riggs, D. S. (1995). Posttraumatic stress disorder following assault: Theoretical considerations and empirical findings. *Current Directions in Psychological Science, 4*(2), 61–65.

Foa, E. B., Riggs, D. S., Massie, E. D., & Yarczower, M. (1995). The impact of fear activation and anger on the efficacy of exposure treatment for posttraumatic stress disorder. *Behavior Therapy, 26,* 487–499.

Foa, E. B., & Rothbaum, B. O. (2001). *Treating the trauma of rape: Cognitive-behavioral therapy for PTSD.* New York: Guilford Press.

Foa, E. B., Rothbaum, B. O., Riggs, D. S., & Murdock, T. B. (1991). Treatment of posttraumatic stress disorder in rape victims: A comparison between cognitive-behavioral procedures and counseling. *Journal of Consulting and Clinical Psychology, 59*(5), 715–723.

Forbes, D., Creamer, M., Bisson, J., Cohen, J., Crow, B., Foa, E., et al. (2010). A guide to guidelines for the treatment of PTSD and related conditions. *Journal of Traumatic Stress, 23*(5), 537–552.

Forbes, D., Creamer, M., Phelps, A., Bryant, R., McFarlane, A., Devilly, G., et al. (2007). Australian guidelines for the treatment of adults with acute stress disorder and post-traumatic stress disorder. *Australian and New Zealand Journal of Psychiatry, 41*(8), 637–648.

Frankl, V. E. (1959). *From death-camp to existentialism: A psychiatrist's path to a new therapy.* Boston: Beacon Press.

French, S. E. (2004). *The code of the warrior: Exploring warrior values past and present.* Lanham, MD: Roman & Littlefield.

Friedman, M. J. (2006). Posttraumatic stress disorder among military returnees from Afghanistan and Iraq. *American Journal of Psychiatry, 163,* 586–593.

Gortner, E., Rude, S. S., & Pennebaker, J. W. (2006). Benefits of expressive writing in lowering rumination and depressive symptoms. *Behavior Therapy, 37*(3), 292–303.

Gray, M., Schorr, Y., Nash, W., Lebowitz, L., Lansing, L., Lang, A., et al. (2012). Adaptive disclosure: An open trial of a novel exposure-based intervention for service members with combat-related psychological stress injuries. *Behavior Therapy, 43*(2), 407–415.

Greenberg, L. S., & Safran, J. D. (1989). Emotion in psychotherapy. *American Psychologist, 44,* 19–29.

Hardy, S. A., & Carlo, G. (2011). Moral identity: What is it, how does it develop, and is it linked to moral action? *Child Development Perspectives, 5*(3), 212–218.

Heinz, K. (1977). *The restoration of the self.* Chicago: University of Chicago Press.

Herman, J. L. (1997). *Trauma and recovery.* New York: Basic Books.

Hoge, C. W., Castro, C. A., Messer, S. C., McGurk, D., Cotting, D. I., & Koffman, R. L. (2004). Combat duty in Iraq and Afghanistan, mental health problems, and barriers to care. *New England Journal of Medicine, 351,* 13–22.

Institute of Medicine. (2007). *Treatment of PTSD: Assessment of the evidence.* Washington, DC: National Academies Press.

Janoff-Bulman, R. (1992). *Shattered assumptions: Towards a new psychology of trauma.* New York: Free Press.

Karlin, B. E., Ruzek, J. I., Chard, K. M., Eftekhari, A., Monson, C. M., Hembree, E. A., et al. (2010). Dissemination of evidence-based psychological treatments for posttraumatic stress disorder in the Veterans Health Administration. *Journal of Traumatic Stress, 23*(6), 663–673.

Keane, T. M., Fairbank, J. A., Caddell, J. M., Zimering, R. T., & Bender, M. E. (1985). A behavioral approach to assessing and treating post-traumatic stress disorder in Vietnam veterans. In C. Figley (Ed.), *Trauma and its wake* (pp. 257–294). Bristol, PA: Routledge.

Keane, T. M., Wolfe, J., & Taylor, K. L. (1987). Post-traumatic stress disorder: Evidence for diagnostic validity and methods of psychological assessment. *Journal of Clinical Psychology, 43*(1), 32–43.

Kohut, H. (1977). *The restoration of the self.* New York: International Universities Press.

Kolb, L. C. (1987). A neuropsychological hypothesis explaining posttraumatic stress disorders. *American Journal of Psychiatry, 144*(8), 989–995.

Kulka, R. A., Schlenger, W. E., Fairbank, J. A., Hough, R. L., Jordan, B. K., Marmar, C. R., et al. (1990). *Trauma and the Vietnam War generation: Report of findings from the National Vietnam Veterans Readjustment Study* (Brunner/Mazel psychosocial stress series). Philadelphia: Brunner/Mazel.

Lambert, M. J., & Barley, D. E. (2002). Research summary on the therapeutic relationship and psychotherapy outcome. In J. C. Norcross (Ed.), *Psychotherapy relationships that work: Therapist contributions and responsiveness to patients* (pp. 17–32). New York: Oxford University Press.

Lannen, P. K., Wolfe, J., Prigerson, H. G., Onelov, E., & Kreicbergs, U. C. (2008). Unresolved grief in a national sample of bereaved parents: Impaired mental and physical health 4 to 9 years later. *Journal of Clinical Oncology, 26*(36), 5870–5876.

Latham, A. E., & Prigerson, H. G. (2004). Suicidality and bereavement: Complicated grief as psychiatric disorder presenting greatest risk for suicidality. *Suicide and Life-Threatening Behaviors, 34,* 350–362.

Lichtenthal, W. G., Cruess, D. G., & Prigerson, H. G. (2004). A case for establishing complicated grief as a distinct mental disorder in DSM-V. *Clinical Psychology Review, 24*(6), 637–662.

Lichtenthal, W. G., Nilsson, M., Kissane, D. W., Breitbart, W., Kacel, E., Jones, E. C., et al. (2011). Underutilization of mental health services among bereaved caregivers with prolonged grief disorder. *Psychiatric Services, 62*(10), 1225–1229.

Linehan, M. M. (1993). *Cognitive behavioral treatment of borderline personality disorder.* New York: Guilford Press.

Litz, B. T. (2014). Resilience in the aftermath of war trauma: A critical review and commentary. *Interface Focus, 4*(5).

Litz, B. T., & Bryant, R. A. (2009). Early cognitive-behavioral interventions for adults. In E. B. Foa, T. M. Keane, M. J. Friedman, & J. A. Cohen (Eds.), *Effective treatments for PTSD: Practice guidelines from the International Society for Traumatic Stress Studies* (2nd ed., pp. 117–135). New York: Guilford Press.

Litz, B. T., & Schlenger, W. (2009). PTSD in service members and new veterans of the Iraq and Afghanistan wars: A bibliography and critique. *PTSD Research Quarterly, 20*(1), 1–8.

Litz, B. T., Steenkamp, M. M., & Nash, W. P. (2014). Resilience and recovery in the military. In L. Zoellner & N. Feeney (Eds.), *Facilitating resilience and recovery following traumatic events* (pp. 113–133). New York: Guilford Press.

Litz, B. T., Stein, N., Delaney, E., Lebowitz, L., Nash, W. P., Silva, C., et al. (2009). Moral injury and moral repair in war veterans: A preliminary model and intervention strategy. *Clinical Psychology Review, 29*(8), 695–706.

Maercker, A., Brewin, C. R., Bryant, R. A., Cloitre, M., Ommeren, M., Jones, L. M., et al. (2013). Diagnosis and classification of disorders specifically associated with stress: Proposals for ICD-11. *World Psychiatry, 12*(3), 198–206.

Martz, E., & Lindy, J. (2010). Exploring the trauma membrane concept. In E. Martz (Ed.), *Trauma rehabilitation after war and conflict* (pp. 27–54). New York: Springer.

McCann, I. L., & Pearlman, L. A. (1990). Vicarious traumatization: A framework for understanding the psychological effects of working with victims. *Journal of Traumatic Stress, 3*(1), 131–149.

McDonagh, A., Friedman, M., McHugo, G., Ford, J., Sengupta, A., Mueser, K., et al. (2005). Randomized trial of cognitive-behavioral therapy for chronic posttraumatic stress disorder in adult female survivors of childhood sexual abuse. *Journal of Consulting and Clinical Psychology, 73*, 515–524.

Mental Health Advisory Team (MHAT IV). (2006). *Operation Iraqi Freedom 05–07.* Washington, DC: Office of the Surgeon Multinational Force–Iraq, and Office of the Surgeon General, U.S. Army Medical Command.

Mental Health Advisory Team V (MHAT V). (2008). *Operation Iraqi Freedom 06–08.* Washington, DC: Office of the Surgeon, Multinational Force–Iraq, and Office of the Surgeon General, U.S. Army Medical Command.

Merrill, L. L., Newell, C. E., Thomsen, C. J., Gold, S. R., Milner, J. S., Koss, M. P., et al. (1999). Childhood abuse and sexual revictimization in a female Navy recruit sample. *Journal of Traumatic Stress, 12*(2), 211–225.

Mowrer, O. H. (1960). Two-factor learning theory: Versions one and two. In O. H. Mowrer (Ed.), *Learning theory and behavior* (pp. 63–91). New York: Wiley.

Nash, W. P. (1998). Information gating: An evolutionary model of personality function and dysfunction. *Psychiatry, 61*, 46–60.

Nash, W. P. (2007). Combat/operational stress adaptations and injuries. In C. R. Figley & W. P. Nash (Eds.), *Combat stress injury: Theory, research, and management* (pp. 33–64). New York: Routledge.

National Collaborating Centre for Mental Health (U.K.). (2005). *Post-traumatic stress disorder: The management of PTSD in adults and children in primary and secondary care.* Leicester, UK: Gaskell.

Norrholm, S. D., Jovanovic, T., Olin, I. W., Sands, L. A., Karapanou, I., Bradley, B., et al. (2011). Fear extinction in traumatized civilians with posttraumatic stress disorder: Relation to symptom severity. *Biological Psychiatry, 69*(6), 556–563.

Paul, L. A., Gros, D. F., Strachan, M., Worsham, G., Foa, E. B., & Acierno, R. (2014). Prolonged exposure for guilt and shame in a veteran of Operation Iraqi Freedom. *American Journal of Psychotherapy, 68*(3), 277–286.

Pitman, R. K., Orr, S. P., Altman, B., Longpre, R. E., Poiré, R. E., Macklin, M. L., et al. (1996). Emotional processing and outcome of imaginal flooding therapy in Vietnam veterans with chronic posttraumatic stress disorder. *Comprehensive Psychiatry, 37*(6), 409–418.

Pivar, I. L., & Field, N. P. (2004). Unresolved grief in combat veterans with PTSD. *Journal of Anxiety Disorders, 18*(6), 745–755.

Pressfield, S. (2011). *The warrior ethos.* Los Angeles: Black Irish Entertainment LLC.

Prigerson, H., & Jacobs, S. (2001). Traumatic grief as a distinct disorder: A rationale, consensus criteria, and a preliminary empirical test. In M. Stroebe, R. Hansson, W. Stroebe, & H. Schut (Eds.), *Handbook of bereavement research:*

Consequences, coping, and care (pp. 613–645). New York: American Psychological Association.

Prigerson, H., Maciejewski, P. K., & Rosenheck, R. (2001). Combat trauma: Trauma with highest risk of delayed onset and unresolved posttraumatic stress disorder symptoms, unemployment, and abuse among men. *Journal of Nervous and Mental Disease, 189*, 99–108.

Prigerson, H. G., Bierhals, A. J., Kasl, S. V., Reynolds, C., Shear, M. K., Day, N., et al. (1997). Traumatic grief as a risk factor for mental and physical morbidity. *American Journal of Psychiatry, 154*, 616–623.

Prigerson, H. G., Bierhals, A. J., Kasl, S. V., Reynolds, C. F., III, Shear, M. K., Newsom, J. T., et al. (1996). Complicated grief as a disorder distinct from bereavement-related depression and anxiety: A replication study. *American Journal of Psychiatry, 153*, 1484–1486.

Prigerson, H. G., Frank, E., Kasl, S. V., Reynolds, C. F., Anderson, B., Zubenko, G. S., et al. (1995). Complicated grief and bereavement-related depression as distinct disorders: Preliminary empirical validation in elderly bereaved spouses. *American Journal of Psychiatry, 152*(1), 22–30.

Prigerson, H. G., Horowitz, M. J., Jacobs, S. C., Parkes, C. M., Aslan, M., Goodkin, K., et al. (2009). Prolonged grief disorder: Psychometric validation of criteria proposed for DSM-V and ICD-11. *PLoS Medicine, 6*(8), e1000121.

Rauch, S. A., Defever, E., Favorite, R., Duroe, A., Garrity, C., Martis, B., et al. (2009). Prolonged exposure for PTSD in a Veterans Health Administration PTSD clinic. *Journal of Traumatic Stress, 22*, 60–64.

Rauch, S. A., Smith, E., Duax, J., & Tuerk, P. (2013). A data-driven perspective: Response to commentaries by Maguen and Burkman (2013) and Steenkamp et al. (2013). *Cognitive and Behavioral Practice, 20*(4), 480–484.

Ready, D. J., Thomas, K. P., Worley, V., Backscheider, A. G., Harvey, L. A. C., Baltzell, D., et al. (2008). A field test of group exposure therapy with 102 veterans with war-related posttraumatic stress disorder. *Journal of Traumatic Stress, 21*, 150–157.

Resick, P. A., Monson, C. M., & Chard, K. M. (2014). *Cognitive processing therapy: Veteran/military version: Therapist and patient materials manual.* Washington, DC: Department of Veterans Affairs.

Resick, P. A., & Schnicke, M. K. (1992). Cognitive processing therapy for sexual assault victims. *Journal of Consulting and Clinical Psychology, 60*(5), 748–756.

Resick, P. A., & Schnicke, M. K. (1993). *Cognitive processing therapy for rape victims: A treatment manual* (Vol. 4). Newbury Park, CA: Sage.

Rosen, C. S., Chow, H. C., Finney, J. F., Greenbaum, M. A., Moos, R. H., Sheikh, J. I., et al. (2004). VA practice patterns and practice guidelines for treating posttraumatic stress disorder. *Journal of Traumatic Stress, 17*(3), 213–222.

Rosen, L. N., & Martin, L. (1996). The measurement of childhood trauma among male and female soldiers in the U.S. Army. *Military Medicine, 161*(6), 342–345.

Roth, S., & Cohen, L. J. (1986). Approach, avoidance, and coping with stress. *American Psychologist, 41*(7), 813–819.

Schnurr, P. P., Friedman, M. J., Engel, C. C., Foa, E. B., Shea, M. T., Chow, B. T., et al. (2007). Cognitive behavioral therapy for posttraumatic stress disorder in women: A randomized controlled trial. *Journal of the American Medical Association, 8,* 820–830.

Schnurr, P. P., Friedman, M. J., Foy, D. W., Shea, M. T., Hsieh, F. Y., Lavori, P. W., et al. (2003). Randomized trial of trauma-focused group therapy for post-traumatic stress disorder: Results from a Department of Veterans Affairs cooperative study. *Archives of General Psychiatry, 60*(5), 481–489.

Schultz, J. R., Bell, K. M., Naugle, A. E., & Polusny, M. A. (2006). Child sexual abuse and adulthood sexual assault among military veteran and civilian women. *Military Medicine, 171*(8), 723–728.

Shanker, T. (2011, May 21). At West Point, a focus on trust. *The New York Times,* p. A21.

Shear, K., Frank, E., Houch, P. R., & Reynolds, C. F. (2005). Treatment of complicated grief: A randomized controlled trial. *Journal of the American Medical Association, 293,* 2601–2608.

Smith, E. R., Duax, J. M., & Rauch, S. (2013). Perceived perpetration during traumatic events: Clinical suggestions from experts in prolonged exposure therapy. *Cognitive and Behavioral Practice, 20*(4), 461–470.

Steenkamp, M., & Litz, B. T. (2013). Psychotherapy for military-related post-traumatic stress disorder: Review of the evidence. *Clinical Psychology Review, 33*(1), 45–53.

Steenkamp, M., Litz, B. T., Gray, M., Lebowitz, L., Nash, W., Conoscenti, L., et al. (2011). A brief exposure-based intervention for service members with PTSD. *Cognitive and Behavioral Practice, 18,* 98–107.

Steenkamp, M., Nash, W., Lebowitz, L., & Litz, B. (2013). How best to treat deployment-related guilt and shame: Commentary on Smith, Duax, and Rauch (2013). *Cognitive and Behavioral Practice, 20*(4), 471–475.

Stein, N. R., Mills, M. A., Arditte, K., Mendoza, C., Borah, A. M., Resick, P. A., et al. (2012). A scheme for categorizing traumatic military events. *Behavior Modification, 36*(6), 787–807.

Stroebe, M., Schut, H., & Boerner, K. (2010). Continuing bonds in adaptation to bereavement: Toward theoretical integration. *Clinical Psychology Review, 30*(2), 259–268.

Suris, A., & Lind, L. (2008). Military sexual trauma: A review of prevalence and associated health consequences in veterans. *Trauma, Violence, and Abuse, 9*(4), 250–269.

van der Kolk, B. A., Roth, S., Pelcovitz, D., Sunday, S., & Spinazzola, J. (2005). Disorders of extreme stress: The empirical foundation of a complex adaptation to trauma. *Journal of Traumatic Stress, 18*(5), 389–399.

Weathers, F. W., Litz, B. T., Herman, D. S., Huska, J. A., & Keane, T. M. (1993, October). *The PTSD Checklist (PCL): Reliability, validity, and diagnostic utility.* Presented at the annual convention of the International Society for Traumatic Stress Studies, San Antonio, TX.

Index

Note: *f* or *t* following a page number indicates a figure or a table.